The Allergy and Asthma Cure

Also by Fred Pescatore, M.D., M.P.H.

Feed Your Kids Well

Thin For Good

The Allergy and Asthma Cure

A Complete 8-Step Nutritional Program

FRED PESCATORE, M.D., M.P.H.

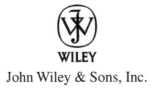

WILEY

John Wiley & Sons, Inc.

Published by John Wiley & Sons, Inc., Hoboken, New Jersey
Published simultaneously in Canada

Limit of Liability/Disclaimer of Warranty: While the publisher and the author have used their best efforts in preparing this book, they make no representations or warranties with respect to the accuracy or completeness of the contents of this book and specifically disclaim implied warranties of merchantability or fitness for a particular purpose. No warranty may be created or extended by sales representatives or written sales materials. The advice and strategies contained herein may not be suitable for your situation. You should consult with a professional where appropriate. Neither the publisher nor the author shall be liable for any loss of profit or any other commercial damages, including but not limited to special, incidental, consequential, or other damages.

For general information about our other products and services, please contact our Customer Care Department within the United States at (800) 762-2974, outside the United States at (317) 572-3993 or fax (317) 572-4002.

Wiley also publishes its books in a variety of electronic formats. Some content that appears in print may not be available in electronic books. For more information about Wiley products, visit our web site at www.wiley.com.

Library of Congress Cataloging-in-Publication Data:

Pescatore, Fred, date.
    The allergy and asthma cure : a complete 8-step nutritional program / Fred Pescatore.
        p. ; cm.
    Includes bibliographical references and index.
    ISBN 978-0-471-21468-7 (cloth)
    ISBN 978-0-470-27541-2 (paper)
    1. Food allergy—Diet therapy. 2. Asthma—Diet therapy. 3. Allergy—Alternative treatment. 4. Asthma—Alternative treatment.
        [DNLM: 1. Food Hypersensitivity—diagnosis—Popular Works. 2. Food Hypersensitivity—Diet therapy—Popular Works. 3. Asthma—diagnosis—Popular Works. 4. Asthma—Diet therapy—Popular Works. 5. Candid—immunology—Popular Works. 6. Dietary Supplements—Popular Works. WD 310 P473a 2003] I. Title.
    RC588.D53 P47 2003
    616.97'5'0654—dc21—dc21
                                            2002014024

10 9 8 7 6 5 4 3

This book is dedicated to SHF,
without whom I could accomplish nothing.

Author's Note

The information in this book reflects the author's experience and is not intended to replace the advice of your own personal physician. It is not the intent of the author to diagnose or prescribe treatment. The intent is only to help you breathe better through a unique program that you may never have tried before, in conjunction with your own personal physician. Only your personal physician can determine if this program is suitable for you, depending on your personal medical history. You should never attempt to decrease your use of medication that has been prescribed for you without first contacting the physician who prescribed it. In addition to regular checkups and supervision, any questions or symptoms that may arise should be addressed to your own personal physician.

This book is not meant to serve as a replacement for your personal physician. Rather, it should be used as an adjunct to what you have been doing in your quest to breathe easier and suffer from fewer symptoms associated with your allergies or asthma.

In the event you use this information without your doctor's approval, you are prescribing for yourself, and the publisher and the author assume no responsibility.

Contents

PART III   The Allergy and Asthma Cure
Nutritional Program

PART IV   The Allergy and Asthma Cure
Meal Plans and Recipes

Recipes

Acknowledgments

This book would not have been written had it not been for the inspiration of the following people:

PG, AB, AG, and AG—for believing that this could help countless other people and forcing me to commit this to paper

EM and GJ—for believing in this project and getting it started

HE—for her amazing recipes

DC—for always being there

TM—for being the best editor one could hope for

And to all the amazing patients who put their trust and confidence in me that I will help them get well. They are the best source of inspiration any doctor could ever hope for.

I couldn't have done this without all of you. Thanks.

Introduction

Is it possible to have a cure for allergies and asthma? Conventional medicine would tell you no. However, in my practice, I have been able to rid or at the very least reduce many of my patients' use of multiple medications they once relied on to treat their allergies and asthma. Could this be considered a cure? Possibly. The one thing I do know is that this would certainly be good news for the millions of people who have ever had to get rid of a pet, stay indoors, or feel miserable for an entire season because of their allergies, or who suffer with asthma—a chronic and life-threatening condition.

I would like to tell you a story about a little boy who was grossly overweight. This didn't bother him so much. He was troubled by the fact that he was unable to breathe well because he seemed to be allergic to everything and had asthma. He was frightened to go swimming, and wouldn't ever play outside in the cold weather because this triggered his asthma attacks. He couldn't play sports in school because he couldn't run and keep up with the other kids. He often had nightmares about not being able to breathe. The dream he had most often was that he was drowning and gasping for air, and he would often wake up screaming for his mother. Sometimes these dreams would trigger an asthma attack and he would spend the rest of the night awake, even after the medicine had its effect, fearful that this would happen again.

This lasted for years and took a toll on his physical as well as his emotional health. His asthma wasn't even that bad. He only needed to use his inhalers as needed and was not placed on any preventive medication except antihistamines during allergy season. As he got older, his allergies decreased to twice per year — in the spring for two months, and again in the fall, for two to three months. He became used to feeling miserable almost six months of the year, and felt thankful that it was only half the year.

As the years went by, his allergies and asthma became things he learned to live with. Physically. Emotionally, his biggest fear became not being able to breathe. As this overweight child approached his teen years, he decided to do something about his appearance, and, by his own volition, he went on a diet to lose weight. He was quite successful and managed to lose sixty pounds. After a certain number of fasting days, he decided to resume eating again, but eliminated all sugar, most bread, and basically ate hamburgers and salads with olive oil dressing. To his utter amazement, his allergies and asthma went away. He was stunned. He did not intend for that to happen; he was entering puberty and wanted to look good. He threw away his inhalers and antihistamines and never looked back.

That little boy was me.

In my practice, probably because of my background, I treat many patients with allergies and asthma. I am almost always successful by using a combination of dietary modifications and nutritional supplements. One of my success stories came to see me for a routine follow-up visit and to basically tell me how well he was doing, now two years into the program. He was renting a house in the country and wanted to tell me that he hadn't needed to use his inhaler, not even once. Prior to starting this program, he had always needed his inhaler because he suffered from allergies to grasses and pollens, and the country always made his asthma symptoms worse. He was still stunned by his progress two years into the program. He told me that he often visits the allergy- and asthma-related Web sites and chat rooms simply to tell the story of his success. It seemed to him that everyone was clamoring to know what he had done and he felt bad because he was dispensing medical advice without being a doctor, but he couldn't help himself because he wanted others to do as well as he did. He begged me to write a book on the subject so that more than just his friends and family could benefit from the work I do.

The link between allergies and asthma has been completely substantiated. It is very hard to discuss one without the other. Up to 38 percent of patients with allergies have been diagnosed with asthma, and 78 percent of all those diagnosed with asthma have allergies. The two are diagnosed simultaneously in about 25 percent of all patients. Not only do these two diseases coexist, they may even cause each other due to their underlying mechanisms. This is why it is so important to find a cure, not just a temporary alleviation of symptoms.

The number of people who suffer from allergies has been increasing dramatically in the past few decades. It is now to the point where the majority of us suffer from allergies in some way at some time in our lives. A total of 30 percent of all adults and 40 percent of children suffer from hay fever, or allergic rhinitis, as it is officially called, which is characterized by nasal congestion and itchy eyes.

Allergies can strike at any time, usually without warning. People may go most of their lives without any allergies and then develop them, or they may suffer their entire lives. Once one allergy develops, the person is usually susceptible to more.

There has to be a cause. Some possible theories include the amount of exercise, or lack thereof, that people get, and the increase in obesity rates as causes of allergies—and asthma, too. Also, airborne pollutants, growing dust mite populations, and poor ventilation are all contributing to this growing problem. Allergies are now the most common chronic disease in North America and are more prevalent than heart disease or diabetes. Anyone who suffers from asthma can tell you that an attack is probably one of the most frightening experiences. As a physician, I can tell you that it is the most life-threatening of the common respiratory conditions. I wanted to be able to do something to help people through these serious times.

Asthma is considered an epidemic of its own, with the number of people with asthma more than doubling since 1980, to more than 17 million people in the United States—about 7.2 percent of the population. The number of children in the U.S. with asthma is 4.8 million. This is a 75 percent increase from 1980 through 1994, the last year for which figures are available. Currently, asthma rates are higher among blacks than among whites and persons of other races. The prevalence of asthma decreases with increasing family income, and women have higher rates of asthma than men.

Most people, including those afflicted with asthma, do not even realize that it can be, and is, life-threatening. Despite the fact that there are more conventional treatments available than ever before, the death rate from asthma has more than doubled since 1980—from 8.2 per 100,000 cases to 17.9 per 100,000 cases in 1995. In fact, more than 5,000 Americans died and there were in excess of 500,000 hospitalizations from this disease in 2001.

What makes this even worse is that more children than ever before are dying. Those at greatest risk are boys, blacks, and urban children. Asthma is the number one serious illness among children in North America.

No one is willing to admit why the number of people with asthma increases dramatically each year. It is something we just don't know. Science doesn't even know how asthma takes hold in your body and why it progresses the way it does. However, there are some theories. For one, there is a strong association between the ozone levels in smog and the severity of asthma. Another theory blames indoor air pollution with its many allergens, simply because more people are spending more time indoors than previously. In addition to the amount of time we spend indoors, our environments are more sealed than previously. So not only are we exposed to more indoor allergens, but also the allergens that are propagated in the cooling system, such as molds, and in the heating system, such as dust mites, are more efficiently exposed to us because of an improvement in insulation.

Still another theory proposes that the increase in asthma is because we live in cleaner, more sanitary conditions than in earlier times. Improved household hygiene, vaccinations, and the use of antibiotics have made us relatively free of disease-causing viruses and bacteria. This has allowed our immune system to fall asleep on the job and not to learn everything it needs to learn—predisposing us to allergies and asthma. Another facet of this same theory holds that those with multiple older siblings and those in day care experience decreased asthma prevalence and suffer fewer allergies, because without a daily dose of germs in the first few months and years of life, a child's immune system doesn't learn the valuable lessons it needs to stay in proper fighting shape. Farm animals, pets, and exposure to dust as small children have all been shown to protect your child from developing allergies. In one study, children who grew up on farms were about 40 percent less likely to have asthma and 50 percent less likely to develop allergies.

The rise in the number of people with asthma has been noted in other countries as well, including Canada, Great Britain, France, Denmark, and Germany. This is a global problem, but the traditional medical community is unwilling to look for a cure because the treatment of asthma is an $11 billion per year industry worldwide. More and more drugs are prescribed for patients, yet increasing numbers of people still suffer and continue to die from this disease each year. Most people with asthma or allergies are relieved when they finally find a series of medications that enables them to breathe, not suffer, and often don't wish to take a chance on something new.

The cure in this book has proven so remarkable for my patients that I think you are going to be convinced to take the plunge. It is possible to find ways other than drugs to relieve the symptoms and get to the underlying cause or causes of these allergy and asthma attacks. This book explains the approach I use with my patients. I use a complementary medical approach, combining the best aspects of traditional and alternative medicine.

Asthma, allergies, eczema, hives, sinus difficulties, and other allergic diseases have similar origins and hence similar treatments. While conventional medicine would lead you to believe they are unrelated, that is just not true. I have believed for years that they are all related to an overgrowth of a very common organism found in every one of us in our digestive tracts: *Candida albicans*.

Candida is a fungus that grows in our bodies. It is naturally present throughout our gastrointestinal system. It is normally kept under control by the good, beneficial bacteria that also live in our digestive tracts. When we take too many courses of antibiotics, candida can overgrow, and when it does, we get many of the symptoms that we are talking about in this book: wheezing; coughing; sinus irritation;

nasal irritation; itchy, watery eyes; and difficulty breathing. These symptoms sound very similar to the symptoms of allergies and asthma, don't they? By eliminating candida, we can start to control our symptoms.

The patients with asthma and allergies who come to see me want relief desperately and want to get off their medications. They do not like the side effects of their prescription drugs. It makes them gain weight, feel jittery or spaced out, and decreases their concentration—and that is just in the short term. I am not going to claim that this program will cure everyone of their allergies and asthma. I can claim that many people who follow my advice can decrease significantly the amount of medications they use daily and be able to enjoy aspects of their lives they thought they would have to do without. The program has been proven by my clinical experience to be safe, effective, and easy to follow.

This book will provide you with an eight-step program—a modern prescription for health. I look at health with a multilevel approach. One should start with proper nutrition—the cornerstone of good health—then add a layer of nutritional supplements specifically targeted toward your symptoms and underlying condition, and then lastly add the finishing touches of cleaning up your environment.

The 75 million people in the United States who suffer from allergies, sinusitis, and asthma want a cure. Modern medicine has been unable or unwilling to provide this cure. Hopefully this book will help you, a sufferer from one or more of these conditions, to do something to fight back and take control of your breathing and your health. This program has helped me and many of my patients of all ages to say good-bye to breathlessness, wheezing, and many other symptoms that plagued them for years. I sincerely hope that it does the same for all of you.

PART I

Allergies and Asthma: A Traditional Approach

1

Understanding and Diagnosing Allergies

Jeffrey, a thirty-five-year-old man, came to see me because he had severe seasonal allergies. They were worse in the spring and fall. He had a high-powered job and was unable to perform well at those times. He had marked difficulty breathing and often ended up with chest colds and on oral steroid medications. He felt he had no choice because it was the only way he could breathe. In addition, he was on two different asthma medications, including an inhaled steroid. It got so bad during allergy season that he was using medications around the clock. He was very worried.

Jeffrey was very concerned that his allergies were slowly getting worse over time. And he couldn't understand why his asthma suddenly seemed to be getting worse. He had had asthma since he was a child and allergies since he was a teenager, and he thought he knew how to handle these conditions. He felt they were now out of control, and he was angry and ready to get to the bottom of these problems.

I performed a food sensitivity test, and I tested for candida antibodies, among other, more routine blood tests. I found he had many food sensitivities—almost more than I had ever seen, and his candida antibodies were very high. I explained that anyone who used steroids, especially oral ones, would have a high candida level. I was also certain that he had a condition called leaky gut evidenced by his many food sensitivities.

I explained to him that asthma and allergies were very tightly connected. That would explain why his allergies triggered the worsening of his asthma symptoms. To treat his allergies and his asthma, we eliminated from his diet the candida and foods to which he was sensitive, and placed him on an oral supplement program. By the fall, he was symptom-free and made it though that first season without any problems. He never needed to be on oral steroids, and his breathing had never been better. After that first true test, we then decreased the amounts of all of his other medications, and he made it symptom-free through the next spring, his first without drugs. He was thrilled, and he continues to do well to this day.

The food sensitivity test and the candida test, along with an oral nutritional supplement program, are the cornerstones of my cure. However, before we get to that, let's examine what allergies and asthma really are.

How Allergy Works

An allergy can be broadly defined as an abnormal, adverse, physical reaction of the body to certain substances known as allergens. It is usually referred to as a hypersensitive state because those who suffer from an allergy usually react to quantities of the allergen that leave most people unharmed.

The process of how this allergen can cause a problem in the body involves the immune system. Most allergic individuals will develop an excess of the antibody IgE when exposed to an allergen. The IgE antibodies then attach to mast cells (a component of your immune system), and the mast cells cause histamines and leukotrienes to be released from certain other cells, causing the disturbing allergic reactions. This is your immune system doing its job, but in this case, it overreacts.

Allergy attacks also may occur through a non-IgE-mediated response. This mechanism is less clear from a scientific point of view, but no less irritating. The food sensitivity test measures sensitivities not related to IgE. Candida antibodies do not measure the IgE response. Certain bacteria or foods can create antigen-antibody complexes that lodge themselves in the lungs in this instance, and cause chronic inflammation, without involving IgE at all.

I mention this because most of the commonly available allergy tests search for an IgE response. If the traditional tests are negative, your doctor will tell you that you don't have any allergies. This is not necessarily true.

Allergy Types

There are almost as many types of allergies as there are allergy sufferers. They are usually classified according to what causes them, or the symptoms they cause. Allergens may cause a reaction in several ways: inhalation, injection, ingestion, or through skin contact. Allergic reactions can involve any part of the body but most frequently affect the nose, eyes, lungs, and skin.

Allergies That Are Defined by What Causes Them

1. *Inhalant allergy,* such as from pollen or dust
2. *Infectious allergy,* with symptoms made worse by a cold or flu
3. *Insect allergy,* usually from the bite of a particular insect
4. *Drug allergy,* which can be quite serious and may result in anaphylaxis—a life-threatening condition
5. *Physical agent allergy,* such as an allergy to cold, heat, or exercise
6. *Contact allergy,* such as to latex, household chemicals, or newsprint
7. *Food allergy,* including anything that you could ingest that is not a poison; it is different from a food sensitivity. Food allergies are generally severe and will cause a noticeable reaction

Allergies That Are Defined by Their Symptoms

1. *Allergic rhinitis or hay fever,* the most common form of allergy
2. *Eczema*

3. *Hives,* also known as chronic urticaria
4. *Skin rashes,* including rashes that are not included in any other grouping
5. *Rosacea*
6. *Anaphylactic shock*

For the majority of the listed allergies, with the exception of anaphylactic shock, drug allergy, and true food allergy, I have been able to help patients achieve close to total resolution of their symptoms through the program outlined in this book.

Allergic Rhinitis or Hay Fever

Although the name may be a misnomer since this rarely produces a fever and hay has nothing to do with it, hay fever affects millions of people. Most people are allergic to pollens, and that is why the symptoms are seasonal. The most common offenders are trees, grasses, and ragweed. The timing of the symptoms is variable due to where you live. Other common offenders are weeds, dust mites, and mold spores.

The symptoms of allergic rhinitis can make us very uncomfortable. Nasal congestion is usually the most troubling of the symptoms—it can affect our speech and give us a dry mouth. Other symptoms include a runny nose, and swelling and inflammation of the mucus membranes. This inflammation causes sneezing, itchy eyes, itchy and scratchy throat, and loss of smell and taste, all of which can make life miserable for a hay fever sufferer. Most people also get a clear mucus drainage that leads them to blow their nose all day and to get a red nose from the irritation.

Allergic rhinitis symptoms also include the following characteristics:

* intermittent symptoms that are either seasonal, food-related, environmental, or emotionally triggered
* symptoms are relieved with antihistamines, food elimination, environmental elimination, or stress reduction techniques
* symptoms are persistent or perennial
* postnasal drip, sore throat, cough, hoarseness, wheezing or difficulty breathing, and/or skin rash

- dark circles under the eyes
- symptoms are usually preceded by a personal or family history of allergies, eczema, or asthma

Eczema

This is one of the most common skin conditions. Eczema as an infant is a strong indicator of asthma risk as a child or an adult. Not all eczema sufferers as infants will go on to suffer from asthma, but almost all asthma sufferers will have had eczema when they were infants. How many of you right now are wondering if you had eczema when you were a baby? Call your mom and ask her.

Eczema is a rash that is most often accompanied by severe itching. It usually begins within the first year of life as a facial rash. Recently, I have been seeing this in adults with no history of having had it. When it begins in adults, the lesions can appear anywhere, but most occur on the insides of the elbows, and on the backs of the knees, neck, ankles, wrists, and hands. Contact eczema occurs when you touch something you are allergic to.

Food Allergy

There are many foods that can cause true allergies. These can be life-threatening and are quite common. A food allergy occurs through an IgE-mediated response similar to what I have previously described. The most common symptoms of a food allergy are vomiting; stomach pain; asthma attack; breathing difficulties; headaches; joint swelling and pain; hives; itchiness; diarrhea; and, in the worst cases, anaphylaxis. Some minor food allergy symptoms can be a tingling sensation in the mouth or a swelling of the tongue.

Some people are so allergic to certain foods that they will get a reaction if the food is simply in the room, or if their skin comes into contact with the food. Sometimes patients may even have reactions to food residue on restaurant tables and chairs. Ninety percent of all food allergies are to milk, peanuts, soy, eggs, nuts such as cashews, almonds, or walnuts (peanuts are actually legumes), shellfish, fish, or wheat. Peanuts, fish, shellfish, and nuts usually cause the most severe reactions.

Peanut allergies are increasingly common, and this is especially important in school-age children because peanuts are in so many foods. It is not just the peanut itself that can cause the allergy but also peanut oil, peanut sauce, and anything that contains peanuts. Peanut oil is so commonly used that it may be one of the ingredients in your food, so check labels. Peanut allergies are usually so severe that if a pot had peanut oil in it prior to your use, a reaction may occur. Peanut allergies are very common, and the reactions tend to be the most severe. Peanuts are responsible for 63 percent of all food-allergy-related deaths.

For this type of severe food allergy, I recommend three things:

1. *Prepare for an emergency.* Should a situation arise where the allergy occurs, you and/or your child should know immediately what to do. In the case of a young child, let the school or sitter know exactly what to do and send written instructions with the child so there is no confusion.
2. *Very careful shopping.* Read food labels very carefully. Know what is in everything that you buy or that your child is buying at school or in a store. If you don't know what is in a particular item and the school or store can't tell you, do not buy it. Always carry a snack for yourself or your child in case there is nothing else available. This especially holds true for airline travel. Never get caught unprepared.
3. *Carry an Epi-pen.* This is a disposable cartridge that carries the drug epinephrine. Learn how to use it, and teach anyone, including your child, in its proper use. This is something you get a prescription for from your doctor.

Diagnosing Your Allergies

Since allergies play such a significant role in lost productivity, increased healthcare costs, and simply making your life miserable, it is important to determine which allergens are responsible for specific diseases, so the proper medical decisions can be made. Allergy testing has serious limitations, and the diagnosis of an allergy to a specific allergen cannot be made on the basis of testing alone. Your history is just as critical to the diagnosis. The basic conventional forms of allergy testing include percutaneous testing, intradermal testing, in vitro antibody testing, and delayed hypersensitivity testing.

Percutaneous Testing

This is the skin prick testing most of us are familiar with. The basic mechanism behind skin testing is the interaction of the injected allergen with specific IgE antibodies on the surface of your skin mast cells. This injection will trigger the release of histamine and the formation of a wheal and flare at the site. A wheal is the swelling you see; a flare is the redness. This reaction usually will occur within fifteen minutes after the allergen is introduced. This test remains the primary diagnostic procedure to determine the cause of allergies in this country.

Most practitioners perform this test on the back of the forearm, the upper arm, or the upper back. The upper back is by far the most sensitive but is not used as often. Certain guidelines should be followed to ensure that the test is done properly. For example, each allergen must be a certain distance apart, never done near the wrist or the elbow, and skin testing should never be performed on sites of active skin flare-ups such as dermatitis or hives.

Your doctor should use both positive and negative controls. A negative control tests the diluent that the allergen is in, to make sure you are not allergic to that rather than to the allergen. A positive control is usually histamine itself, to ensure that your body's immune system is giving an adequate response.

The prick test can be performed in patients as young as one month of age, although this is quite rarely done. Allergen skin reactions start to decline in adults after one's twenties, due to decreased skin reactivity to histamine and lower IgE levels. Therefore, if you are older than this when this test is done, you may get many false negative results.

This test is also limited because it measures only a clinically immediate IgE hypersensitivity. If you do not have an IgE-mediated allergy, the test will be negative, and your doctor will tell you that you are not allergic to a certain substance. The test is also dependent on the person performing the test. Such factors as the exact amount of allergen used, the depth and force of the needle, the duration of force, the angle of application, and the stability of the allergen extracts are all variables that can cloud interpretation of the test.

Use of antihistamines should be stopped twenty-four to seventy-two hours prior to taking these tests; use of tricyclic antidepressants and benzodiazepines (Valium and similar substances) need to be stopped for seven to fourteen days beforehand; use of systemic corticosteroids and topical steroids should be stopped up to three weeks prior to any testing. It is believed that nonsteroidal medications such as ibuprofen do not interfere, but I always advise my patients to stop use of these as well. You do not want anything to interfere with the accuracy of your test results. It is better to get a proper test result than one that does not give you the correct information.

Intradermal Testing

This is used when skin prick testing is not deemed sensitive enough to detect the cause of an allergic reaction. This is usually what happens when a patient tests negative on a prick test but has a strong clinical history of symptoms triggered by exposure to a specific allergen. This should also be used in patients for whom skin prick testing is not valid, as in anyone over thirty. However, skin prick testing usually is done first, to avoid a systemic allergic reaction, which may be quite serious.

Intradermal testing is performed through injection of an allergen extract that is diluted a hundred to a thousand times of what would be given in a skin prick test. It is injected into the back of the forearm or on the upper arm. Swelling occurs immediately; changes in the size of the swelling and the redness are measured after twenty minutes.

This test also has limitations because small positive reactions may actually not be reactions, and positive and negative controls must be used so the test is interpreted properly. Despite their many drawbacks, percutaneous testing and interdermal testing are the most widely used conventional allergy tests.

In Vitro Antibody Testing

The first test of this kind was the RAST (radioallergosorbent test). It is a simple blood test that measures the amount of IgE that binds to a specific allergen versus the amount of IgE that doesn't. This test can be used in patients for whom skin testing cannot be performed, such as those who cannot stop taking their medications, those with severe skin conditions, and those who have near-fatal reactions to certain offending substances.

The main disadvantage of this type of test is that there is no uniform method for reporting results, making separate tests not comparable to each other and difficult to use in clinical practice with any certainty. I hardly ever recommend this test because of its lack of useful information.

Delayed Hypersensitivity Testing

Whereas skin prick tests measure IgE immediate hypersensitivity responses, delayed hypersensitivity testing uses patches to measure type 4 delayed hypersensitivity. A clinical example of this involves contact dermatitis. The antigens that cause this type of reaction are found in cosmetics, jewelry, household cleansers, and similar products, as opposed to pollens and foods.

This test is performed by applying various materials to an absorbent pad, which is then placed on your skin, usually your back. The site is then checked at forty-eight and at seventy-two hours after application. A positive response is characterized by redness and swelling. Most of us have taken a test like this such as for tuberculosis—a PPD.

Is Conventional Testing Important?

Conventional testing of allergies remains an important part of any workup in a patient. Most of my patients have already been tested before they come to see me. I just review the testing to ensure that they have been tested correctly. Allergy testing can confirm a reaction to clinically suspected allergens.

If you do undergo allergy testing—and I highly recommend that you do—here are the main points to keep in mind:

1. Percutaneous testing should be done first.
2. Intradermal testing should be done on anyone over thirty or on anyone who tested negative to the percutaneous test, especially if the allergen is highly suspicious.
3. Percutaneous and intradermal testing must be performed and interpreted by an experienced practitioner.

4. In vitro antibody testing (RAST) gives little useful information, so I recommend that you not have it done.
5. If something tests positive, then do everything you can to avoid it—even if it means drastic changes in your life.

Despite their importance in helping to diagnose your problem, these conventional tests usually show positive for the same things in most patients: molds, dust, grasses, pollens, and cats. I would say that most of my patients have had these tests and have been found to be positive to at least one of those five things. That information never did them any good.

While it is true that most of us are allergic to these things, there is something missing in the diagnostic process. I have seen too many patients who eliminate these things from their environment, and still suffer. I believe I have found why this occurs, and that is what this book is about.

Allergens and Asthma

There are many allergens that need to be recognized, and their elimination needs to be addressed for you to feel as good as you want to feel. You will be shocked by how many environmental triggers I am going to mention. Since allergies and asthma are so closely related, I will discuss the long list of allergens in the next chapter.

2

Understanding and Diagnosing Asthma

John, a thirty-seven-year-old man, came to my office because of a problem he had never experienced before. He had come down with a cold or flu and was having difficulty breathing. He thought he had pneumonia. When I listened to his lungs, there were a lot of whistles and high-pitched noises there—he was wheezing. I explained to him that this was common with an upper respiratory infection and that it would go away. Three months later during a wet fall season, John came back to my office with the same shortness of breath—only this time, it happened to him while playing basketball. He was coughing, and he also felt some tightness in his chest. Now he was concerned that he was having a heart attack.

After assuring him that it was not his heart and listening to his lungs and chest, I then knew that he had a new case of asthma, most likely allergy-related. He had never been diagnosed with asthma before, and to the best of his knowledge, had never had these symptoms, and he played basketball a lot. Needless to say, John was shocked when I told him what I thought his diagnosis was.

The diagnosing of a new case of asthma in an adult is a very common occurrence in my office as well as in most other physicians' offices today. There is an epidemic of asthma in our country and around the world. Historically, most people got asthma when they were a child and therefore knew about it as adults. But now a lot of people are getting asthma for the first time as adults, and they want to know why.

Unfortunately, we do not have a good answer to that question. There are many theories, but science has yet to figure out the exact mechanism. A good understanding of the basics will help you try to figure out what you can do to help yourself win this battle against allergies and asthma.

What Is Asthma?

Asthma is the number one chronic respiratory disease in North America. It is a disease of the lungs. The term "asthma" comes from the Greek word for panting. People with asthma pant because, when they are experiencing an attack, the tubes inside their lungs that deliver air, known as bronchi, become inflamed. When this happens, the muscles of the bronchial walls tighten and extra mucus is produced, causing the airway to narrow. The severity of the attack can vary from slight wheezing to life-threatening. These obstructive changes leave very little room for air to get through. Trying to breathe when this is occurring is like trying to breathe with a pillow over your face. To make matters worse, people with asthma get an airway inflammation that produces more mucus, which can lead to even more airway obstruction—a vicious cycle that continues, usually until some medication is administered.

Warning Signs and Symptoms

There do appear to be certain warning signs that often precede a full-blown asthma attack by a few hours. These are:

- Unusual fatigue
- Tight feeling in the chest
- Dry mouth
- Mouth breathing

- Sudden coughing
- Rapid heartbeat
- Anxiety
- Irritability
- Scratchy throat
- Perspiration

These warning signs are the most common, yet I have found them to be quite variable among my patient population. One thing that is common in all people who suffer with asthma is that they can usually tell when they are going to get an attack, although one may still come out of the blue.

Symptoms of an attack also vary. The most common symptoms include difficulty breathing, wheezing upon exhalation, shortness of breath, coughing, constricted chest, or painfully congested lungs. People with asthma can be divided into mild, moderate, and severe cases, depending on their symptoms. Try to see where you fit into these categories.

Mild Asthma

These patients comprise 50 percent of the asthmatic population. They have symptoms only once or twice per year and are generally controlled on "as needed" bronchodilator medications.

Moderate Asthma

Forty percent of all patients with asthma fall into this category. These people have symptoms roughly once per month and some require daily medication to keep their symptoms from getting worse and interfering with their daily life.

Severe Asthma

These cases make up the remainder of patients with asthma. This is the life-threatening form of this condition. However, it should also be remembered that patients in any of the categories can have a life-threatening attack, so please take your condition seriously. The severe types usually require multiple daily medications just to maintain decent control over their breathing. Wheezing and coughing occur most of the time, and these patients usually find it difficult to participate in sporting activities.

How Asthma Works

The pathophysiology (medicalese for how things work on a cellular level) of an asthma attack is quite complex, but I will explain it as best I can. This is a rapidly developing area of scientific research, and the concepts have changed significantly in the past twenty-five years since I was diagnosed with asthma.

Asthma results from the combined effects of allergic airway inflammation and a dysfunction of the muscles in the airway. These are the muscles that cause the constriction to occur. This, along with swelling of the airway, mucus plug formation, and airway remodeling, are the prime causes of the symptoms.

Airway remodeling occurs in someone with a chronic case of asthma over time. The airway will start to take on a different form than it is supposed to have. If the inflammatory effects of asthma are not treated, permanent scarring of the lungs can occur, which can permanently alter airway function.

Swelling of the airway and the formation of mucus take place in two phases—through an immediate and a delayed inflammatory response. This is why attacks often start slowly and build to a frightening crescendo that may lead to hospitalization.

In the immediate phase, there is usually an allergic trigger such as pollen or animal dander. This allergen enters the lungs and comes into contact with the bloodstream. When this occurs, the central figure in this entire process is activated, the CD-4 or T-cell lymphocyte. A subset of these cells, known as the TH-2 cell, is the exact culprit. This white blood cell recognizes this allergen as a pathogen that should not be in the body and sends a message of danger throughout the immune system. This is the body's natural protective mechanism and how our bodies fight off other diseases quite effectively. In asthma, the response triggered is overblown, and that is what causes the problem.

This TH-2 cell then enlists the help of another white blood cell, called the B cell. B cells then make antibodies called IgE, which are finely tuned to recognize the particles of the pollen. The IgE antibodies then latch on to other immune system cells, called mast cells. The mast cells then release a chemical soup of substances known as histamine, leukotrienes, prostaglandins, and thromboxanes. These are the substances that cause the inflammatory responses that lead to the increased blood flow, edema, and constriction of the airway.

In the delayed phase, cytokines are activated, which further prolong the inflammatory response, and these, in turn, activate basophils, eosinophils, lymphocytes, and more mast cells, leading to the prolongation and exacerbation of the attack. And believe me, that is the simple explanation.

Diagnosing Your Asthma

Asthma can affect someone of any age. Medical science has devised a new terminology to distinguish those who have had asthma since they were children and those who began as adults. Those who developed asthma as adults are classified as late-onset asthmatics or LOA.

Regardless of the age of onset, the diagnostic process should include a detailed medical history, chest X ray, lung function tests, and perhaps an examination of the phlegmlike secretions. In addition, allergy tests are usually necessary. As for the complementary medical tests, I order food sensitivity testing, which I think is invaluable, as well as a test for candida.

History

A diagnosis of asthma cannot be made from one test or even a series of tests. It is more a diagnosis by history. That is why it is important to give your doctor a proper history of the following:

1. When do these events occur?
2. Are they triggered by certain things?
3. When did the symptoms first start?

4. How long do the symptoms last?
5. What do you do to make the symptoms better?
6. Is there a certain time of the year when they are worse?

These and many other questions are the cornerstones in obtaining the proper diagnosis.

Chest X ray: This is a simple test, and in patients with asthma it can show hyperinflation. This means that there is too much air in the lungs. However, that is nondiagnostic, and that same picture can be seen in other lung conditions. In newly diagnosed patients it is important to get a chest X ray to make sure there are no other treatable lung conditions that could be causing the same symptoms, such as pneumonia or cancer.

Sputum evaluation: This test examines your sputum and looks for a certain type of white blood cell known as eosinophils. This is the type of cell that increases when there is an allergic response to a trigger.

Complete blood count (CBC): This is a test of the red and white blood cells. We particularly look at eosinophils and total white blood cell count. If the white blood cell count is elevated, this could indicate an infection such as bronchitis or pneumonia, rather than asthma. It is another test to rule out any other underlying causes for your symptoms. If the eosinophil count is increased, your asthma has a strong allergic component.

Pulmonary function tests (PFT): Most people with asthma are familiar with these tests. They involve blowing into a machine to measure the degree of obstruction present.

The simplest of these tests is known as a peak flow rate test and is measured with a peak flow meter. This works by you inhaling as deeply as you can, and then blowing into this meter as hard and as fast as possible. The meter measures the maximum speed with which air can be forced out of the lungs. If your breathing tubes are blocked, the speed is reduced and you get a reduced peak flow rate.

Conventional allergy testing: This includes percutaneous, intra-dermal, in vitro antibody (RAST) testing, and delayed hyper-sensitivity testing, as described in chapter 1.

Diagnosing Childhood Asthma

Since this is a very common childhood disease, it is critical that parents learn to recognize the symptoms of asthma in their children because it may one day save their life.

Fifty to 80 percent of children with asthma will become symptomatic before age five. Since these symptoms can mimic other childhood diseases, such as respiratory infections and foreign-body aspirations, it is important for a parent to recognize these signs.

There are generally six signs to look for to know if your child is troubled with asthma. These include:

1. *Wheezing.* This is a high-pitched, whistling sound usually more pronounced at night as the child exhales. As an attack progresses, the airways become more blocked and the wheezing may stop. This is not a good sign, but an indication that the condition is getting worse. Wheezing also can occur in nasal or sinus infections and in vocal cord dysfunctions, so be careful.
2. *Breathing differences.* Look at your child with his or shirt off, and if you see the soft tissue being sucked in just below the rib cage, this is a bad sign known as retracting respirations. Also see if your child is using the muscles of the neck or abdomen to breathe—another ominous sign.
3. *Labored breathing.* As the airways get blocked, it is more difficult to get air out of the lungs, and this may occur, resulting in prolonged exhalation. Often it is just as difficult to get air out of the lungs as it is to breathe air into the lungs.
4. *Shortness of breath.* The easiest way to see this in children is to notice if they are having difficulty making sentences, sleeping, or running around.
5. *Panting.* The normal breathing rate will increase as your child struggles to get enough oxygen.
6. *Triggers.* Was the event triggered or aggravated by something specific, such as allergens, cold air, or a sporting event?

Important Differentiations

Since it is critical for treatment to know whether you just have allergies or whether you have allergies and asthma, I have put factors to look for in a simple format to help you determine which ailment you have. The symptoms overlap, so don't take this as a definitive test.

Allergy

- Characterized by fatigue, headache, runny nose, stuffy nose, sneezing, postnasal drip, itchy and watery eyes, scratchy throat
- May occur only during specific seasons, or throughout the year
- Specific trigger for the symptoms
- Have over-the-counter medications for allergies been successful?

Asthma

- Characterized primarily by shortness of breath, wheezing, and coughing
- Not a single condition but may be mild, moderate, or severe, and can be intermittent or persistent
- Can be allergic, nonallergic, exercise-induced, drug-induced, or occupational
- Often involves the need to go to a hospital
- Much more serious condition than most allergies; asthma is more often life-threatening

Although I describe various tests, I can't stress enough how important history is. The timing of the symptoms, the length of their duration, and anything that may have precipitated events are critical determinants of proper diagnosis and treatment. If you can't remember specific events—and oftentimes patients can't—write things down.

Since medical visits have become shorter and shorter over time, you have to learn how to make the system work for you. Allergies and asthma take more time to figure out than the average physician has time for in a short visit. Don't allow your doctor to give you medications without first determining what you have.

Allergies and Asthma: The Overlapping Factors

Pam, a forty-three-year-old woman, came into my office because she had been plagued with asthma her entire life. She so desperately wanted to see me because I had helped her friend get off medication and had explained to her why she had asthma and what she could do to get rid of her condition. I went through Pam's entire life and tried to find out where the allergic triggers for her attacks were. This is a very time-consuming process, but worth it if the result is decreasing the amount of medication you take or eliminating it completely. While it will not always be possible to remove all of the allergy triggers from your life, you will be able to eliminate some when you know what they are. Most people don't realize how many things can bring on an asthma attack.

It is impossible to discuss asthma without also discussing allergies. There is a very strong allergic component to asthma, but not everyone with allergies will have asthma. The cure is designed for people with asthma as well as those who suffer from allergies, frequent colds and flus, bronchitis, rhinitis, sinusitis, eczema, hives, psoriasis, and most other inflammatory-based conditions. There is a strong interconnection among these diseases, so everyone should read this entire book.

In most people with asthma, their attack is usually brought on by an allergic reaction to substances commonly inhaled, such as animal dander and pollens. These are called allergens; asthma also may be triggered by certain other things in the air commonly known as irritants.

Allergens and irritants that may trigger an allergy or asthma attack include:

- Aerosol sprays
- Air pollution
- Animal dander
- Certain medications (such as aspirin or ibuprofen)
- Cockroaches
- Cold outdoor temperatures
- Dust mites
- Estrogen
- Exercise

- Foods
- Gastroesophageal reflux disease (GERD) or heartburn
- Heredity
- Molds (indoor and outdoor)
- Obesity
- Perfumes and other chemicals
- Pollens
- Respiratory and sinus infections
- Smoke
- Strong emotions
- Sulfites (preservatives in red wine, beer, dehydrated soups, salad bars, and other foods)
- Thunderstorms
- Viruses

As you can see from this list, there are many allergens and irritants that may trigger an acute attack of allergies or asthma; and this list is by no means exhaustive. It is easy to see why you may be suffering from asthma attacks and allergy symptoms. Let's look at these triggers more closely to see how they may be eliminated from your environment.

- *Aerosol sprays.* These can include substances such as deodorants and household cleaners. It may not be so much the chemical that you are sensitive to but the propellant that shoots the active ingredients out of the can. These can be removed from your environment by switching to nonaerosol varieties.
- *Air pollution.* This is a tough one to avoid, especially if you live in a large, smoggy city. It is believed that ozone in the air is the irritant. In one study performed during the Atlanta Olympics by Michael S. Friedman, M.D., and W. Gerald Teague, M.D., the incidence of asthma attacks in children in Atlanta during the games dropped precipitously due to a large improvement in air quality at that time because of a decrease in driving. Air pollution appears to be a serious trigger for those who suffer from asthma, so try to stay indoors during ozone alert days.
- *Animal dander.* This is controversial. Some studies show this to be a trigger, while others do not show a connection. In a recent study by Thomas A. Platts-Mills, M.D. at the University of Virginia School of Medicine, it was shown that the higher the level of

exposure to cats, the less likely was a child's risk for developing asthma; but, low levels of exposure increased the risk and seemed to trigger an allergic reaction. It was reported in the 2000 National Health and Nutrition Examination that exposure to household pets accounted for an estimated nine hundred thousand excess cases of asthma each year, and possibly hundreds of millions of allergy attacks.

People are not always allergic to an animal's hair or feathers, but to a protein in the animal's saliva, dander, or urine. That is why it is possible to get an asthma or allergy attack even if the animal isn't around. These protein molecules travel silently through the air, and the allergens are present even when the pet isn't; and these particles can remain in the air and on carpets and furniture for weeks or even months after the pet is gone.

Cat allergens can even be found in homes where cats have never lived and in office buildings where animals aren't allowed. This is because cat allergens are particularly sticky and may be carried on clothing from places with cats to other locations, so it is virtually impossible not to be exposed to some level of cat allergen. About 25 percent of asthma sufferers are allergic to cats.

The most effective way to remove the direct cause of this allergen is to remove the offending pet. Since I would never recommend that, you might do better with certain breeds that have hair instead of fur, such as terriers; or try to keep your pet out of your bedroom. Purchase a HEPA (high-efficiency particulate air) filter for your bedroom, a HEPA-equipped vacuum, and eliminate rugs. If you have bare floors, you should frequently damp-mop them with hot water. Cover mattresses and cushions with zippered plastic so the allergens do not come into contact with you while you sleep.

- *Certain medications.* Aspirin or ibuprofen are the most common offenders, but any other nonsteroidal anti-inflammatory drug can produce the same effect. Beta-blockers used in the treatment of heart disease, migraine headaches, and high blood pressure and in drops for glaucoma also can be linked to asthma attacks. Consult your doctor for alternatives to these medications.
- *Cockroaches.* These are primarily implicated in the increased incidence of asthma in those who live in inner city areas, particularly children. One approach to keeping cockroaches out is by

blocking areas that provide an entrance to your home for these creatures, including crevices, wall cracks, windows, woodwork, and floor gaps. Since they like water, be sure to fix and seal all leaky faucets and pipes. They can also be professionally exterminated, or you can use one of the many products sold in supermarkets. Once you've done your best to eliminate the problem, try to prevent them from returning by keeping food in tightly covered containers, and remember to put pet food dishes away after the animal has eaten. Try to always use lidded garbage containers, and wash dishes and countertops with hot, soapy water immediately after use.

Cold outdoor temperature. Any temperature extreme has been known to trigger an attack, but the cold was an especially bad trigger for me when I was a child. I could barely walk a few blocks when the weather was cold without wheezing and having difficulty breathing. I think that is the main reason why today I prefer warm weather.

Dust mites. These are little critters that are microscopic relatives to spiders. Dust mites live in house dust. Their droppings are the most common triggers of perennial allergy and asthma symptoms such as a congested or runny nose; itchy, watery eyes; coughing; and wheezing.

Dust mites prefer bedding, upholstered furniture, carpets, and curtains. One way to control them is to place mattresses, box springs, and pillows in airtight, zippered plastic, or special allergenproof fabric covers. Wash your bedding weekly in hot water heated to at least 130°F. Dust mites are least likely to collect in comforters and pillows made from synthetic fibers and/or covered with allergenproof fabrics, rather than with natural materials such as down feathers or cotton. Substitute wall-to-wall carpets with hardwood floors, tile, or linoleum flooring, if you can. In this way, you can accent the rooms with washable area rugs of natural fibers without exacerbating your symptoms. Clean the floors frequently with a hot, damp mop.

Weekly vacuuming helps, too. Use a vacuum with a HEPA filter or use a double bag on your regular vacuum cleaner so allergens will get trapped rather than pass through the vacuum's exhaust. Lastly, dust mites thrive in higher humidity levels, so a dehumidifier or air conditioner in the summer can maintain relative humidity below 50 percent throughout your home and help to decrease your allergic reaction to these small critters.

* *Estrogen.* According to recent data from the ongoing Nurses' Health Study, estrogen replacement therapy is associated with an 80 percent higher risk of adult-onset asthma in postmenopausal women. The likelihood of developing asthma grew with higher estrogen doses and longer duration of use. For example, women who were on estrogen-replacement for five years increased their likelihood of developing asthma by 90 percent, compared with those who never took estrogen. Those on estrogen for two to five years increased their risk by 60 percent; the figure was 50 percent in women who used estrogen for fewer than two years. Is it any wonder why I have so many female patients complaining of allergies and skin conditions for the first time when they are postmenopausal?

Approximately a third of female patients with asthma will experience deterioration of airway function before or during menses. This is called ovarian asthma and can be severe enough to cause recurrent respiratory failure and even death. Oral contraceptive therapy has been shown to be useful for gaining asthma control in affected patients.

Despite the fact that estrogen replacement can positively affect the risk for osteoporosis and reduce the symptomatology of menopause, there are many risks to these drugs that should be taken into account, including the risk for asthma.

* *Exercise.* This is a very common trigger for an asthma attack. There are some people for whom this is the only trigger, especially kids. I was one of those kids. A study in *Archives of Pediatrics and Adolescent Medicine* showed that taking 2,000 mg of vitamin C prior to exercise significantly reduced asthma-type symptoms.

* *Foods.* There is a very large group of people for whom food will trigger an asthma or allergy attack. The identification of food sensitivities is a mainstay of the allergy and asthma cure; however, some people have very severe food allergies—their throat may close, or they may break out in hives when they eat an offending food. Some people will even start to wheeze, their airways will

significantly constrict, and this can be a life-or-death situation. Learning to avoid certain foods is the way to control this trigger.

⊙ *Gastroesophageal reflux disease (GERD) or heartburn.* This is acid backing up into your esophagus, and it triggers an asthma attack if the acid gets into your lungs. The attack usually occurs at night in bed, because when you lie down, the acid can move more easily up into your lungs. GERD also can cause asthma through stimulation of the nearby vagus nerve.

In a report at the 2001 meeting of the American College of Gastroenterology, it was said that half of all coughing and wheezing episodes in asthma patients are associated with acid reflux. Theophylline and beta-2 agonists, conventional medications used to treat allergies and asthma, can further increase acid reflux—a great example of the treatment causing the disease. Since treatment of GERD with antireflux medications does not significantly reduce the asthmatic episodes, I don't advise taking them. However, try to avoid heavy meals at bedtime and perhaps take your heavier meal at lunchtime, when you are less likely to lie down after eating. Try to eat at least three hours before you go to bed—and that includes snacks. Drinking alcohol or caffeine, but not water, and smoking can make this problem worse.

⊙ *Heredity.* If one of your parents has asthma, you have a 25 percent chance of having it as well. The likelihood for allergies is even higher if your parents suffered from them.

⊙ *Molds (indoor and outdoor).* This is another major trigger for asthma and allergies. The conventional wisdom focuses on indoor molds and outdoor molds. The mold I will primarily be discussing in the cure and what I feel to be the most significant contributor to this problem is internal mold. More about that later, but let's first discuss these molds.

Indoor molds and mildew are found in damp basements and on bathroom walls and windows. It is the black stuff that you see in the crevices of the tile. Mold also can be found in leaky air conditioners and humidifiers, where fresh food is stored, and in garbage pails.

It is the spores the molds send out when they are reproducing that cause the allergic reaction. Molds are microscopic fungi and are some of the most widespread living organisms. Molds are much more numerous than plant pollens.

The indoor molds can be easily defeated with a cleaning solution containing 5 percent bleach and a small amount of detergent. Eliminate the source by promptly repairing and sealing any leaky pipes or roofs. Make sure to regularly empty the water from any dehumidifier, and clean the unit with bleach. All rooms, but especially basements, bathrooms, and kitchens, require ventilation and consistent cleaning to deter regrowth of molds and mildew. Sunshine, which helps keep things dry, also will discourage mold growth.

Outdoor molds are present in the air unless there is snow on the ground. They are most prevalent in shady and damp areas and on decaying leaves. That is why people with asthma and allergies have a worsening of their symptoms in the fall. The highest levels of molds are in coastal areas, which tend to have more moderate temperatures and the least amount of snowfall.

Obesity. There is a direct correlation between body mass index (BMI) and asthma. To figure out your BMI, do the following: (1) Multiply your weight in pounds by 703; (2) square your height in inches; then 3) divide the total in step 1 by the total in step 2. It is considered optimum for your BMI to be 22; and anyone with a BMI under 25 is considered to be at low risk for developing asthma.

As for adults, the case for obesity causing an increased risk for asthma is clear. Research has shown that for people with a BMI greater than 28, they are at a 2.4 times higher risk for developing asthma. They are also at higher risk for developing emphysema, another bad respiratory condition. Women with a BMI greater than 28 are 3.5 times more likely to develop asthma, but men have only a 40 percent increased risk at that BMI range.

This is more important than ever, since 65 percent of all adults are overweight and 28 percent are obese. In children the figures are slightly lower but still alarming. Approximately one in three children is overweight or obese. This is a 54 percent increase since 1967.

One study from a 2001 *American Journal of Respiratory and Critical Care Medicine* showed that for girls, becoming overweight or obese between ages six and eleven increased their risk of developing new asthma symptoms and increased bronchial responsiveness or wheezing during the early adolescent period. Other studies also have shown that being overweight as a child is associated with more severe asthma symptoms and outcomes. Seventy-eight percent of all asthmatics have allergies as well.

Studies have determined that weight loss can improve the pulmonary status of people with asthma, by decreasing the airway obstruction. This is an important determinant because it proves that you can do something to positively affect your asthma if you are overweight. It also proves that you can decrease your risk for contracting asthma if you are not already overweight.

As I bring out in my previous books *Feed Your Kids Well* and *Thin For Good,* diet is a big concern and focus of my practice. A dietary program is a big part of the allergy and asthma cure. The diets in this book are not as detailed as those in my earlier books, but proper nutrition is essential to getting off of your medications. *Perfumes and Other Chemicals.* We live in a world where we are exposed to chemicals hourly. I will briefly mention some of the most common ones here, but keep in mind that it is impossible to live in a totally chemical-free environment.

Latex is commonly found in gloves used by healthcare workers, and in balloons, condoms, tires, elastic waistbands, rubber toys, bottle nipples, and pacifiers, to name a few. In fact, the American College of Allergy, Asthma, and Immunology reports that more than seven million tons of latex were used in products in the United States alone in 2001.

Formaldehyde is found in such everyday things as new fabrics, plastics, decaffeinated coffee, antiperspirants, germicidal and detergent soap, aerosol deodorants, and even ice cream and mouthwashes.

Acetone in nail polish remover; benzyl alcohol; Congo red (a common dye); polyester; isopropyl glycol, in cosmetics and deodorant sprays; toluene; aniline, the dye used in newsprint; and chromium oxydatum, which is used in the ink on dollar bills, have all been found to be allergen triggers.

These are just a few of the many chemicals that we come into contact with every day. Simply try to avoid the most common offenders as they may be a trigger for your allergies or asthma.

* *Pollens.* These cannot be avoided completely because they are found everywhere and in every season. Pollen is produced by weeds, shrubs, grasses, flowers, and trees. Seasonal patterns vary depending on where you live, so it is important to know the pattern in your geographical area. As a general rule of thumb, tree pollens are most prevalent in the spring, grasses are most prevalent in the late spring and summer, and then ragweed is the biggest culprit from late summer until the first frost. In areas of the country that do not experience frost, seasonal allergies can occur all year long.
* *Respiratory and sinus infections.* I list these together because they are very similar in their effect on the person with asthma. This category includes viruses such as the common cold and the flu, and bacterial infections such as sinusitis, rhinitis, and bronchitis.

  Rhinitis is associated with a five times higher risk of asthma onset. Chronic sinusitis is directly related to the severity of lower airway disease because the nasal secretions irritate the mucosa of the surrounding tissues and cause further inflammation and worsening of the symptoms. The program outlined in this book will help with those conditions, too.
* *Smoke.* Smoke includes tobacco and wood smoke and other airborne pollutants. Although many of us love the smell of a woodburning stove or fire, it can be a real irritant to those with allergies or asthma. Wood burning can cause a large increase in the amount of carbon monoxide and other particles in the air.

  Cigarette smoke contains dozens of potentially irritating chemicals and pollutants. Indoor smoking can increase levels of carbon monoxide, formaldehyde, nitrogen dioxide, acrolein, hydrocarbons, hydrogen cyanide, and many other toxic substances. If you suffer from allergies or asthma, do not smoke, and avoid secondhand smoke as much as you can.
* *Strong Emotions.* Allergies and asthma, especially skin exacerbations, can be made worse by stress and anxiety. This is believed to occur because of a change in normal breathing patterns—making breathing more shallow with decreasing levels of carbon dioxide, which can cause you to hyperventilate. Learning to control stress through stress management techniques could help.
* *Sulfites.* These are very common food preservatives and prevent the browning and discoloration of foods that may occur at room

temperature. They are found in salad bars in many restaurants and delis. They are primarily used to preserve red wine, beer, raw potatoes, fresh vegetables, and dehydrated soups. Sulfites also are in many inhaled asthma medications. Try to avoid food that is not freshly prepared, and red wine.

- *Thunderstorms.* Several researchers have found that due to the way that the air circulates during these storms, asthma attacks may be triggered because the downdrafts of air sweep up pollen grains and particles and concentrate them at ground level. This trigger is especially prevalent during the late spring and summer, when pollen counts are at their highest, and so are thunderstorms.
- *Viruses.* These are some of the most abundant organisms on the planet. The common cold and the flu are two such examples that we all suffer from. These organisms can cause you to have difficulty breathing and nasal congestion all by themselves. People who are prone to asthma would likely have their condition worsen when they come into contact with a virus.

By knowing what may cause an attack, you can be better prepared for it, and hopefully be able to avoid the trigger. Part of my cure is the removal of many of these triggers. By doing this, you can begin to rid your body of inflammation and then the drugs. A recent study in the medical journal *Pediatrics* said it best: Reducing the exposure of a child with asthma to indoor allergy risks could result in a 44 percent decline in asthma cases among older children and adolescents. Wouldn't it be great to reduce your asthma attacks by that much just by reducing your exposure to certain allergens? That should be part of any allergy and asthma cure.

3

Conventional Therapies for the Treatment of Allergies

When Drew, a thirty-eight-year-old stockbroker, came to see me he was stressed out because it was allergy season again and he couldn't find an effective medication that didn't leave him with some unpleasant side effect. As he got older, he found that he was seemingly becoming increasingly allergic to things and needed more and more medication just to be able to breathe. It was affecting more than his job performance; both his physical and his sexual activity were being curtailed because he just didn't feel well. He was moving up the ranks in his company and really needed to be at his peak; he couldn't afford to feel anything but his best. He came to me because I had helped one of his friends with a weight issue and he wanted to see if there was anything I could do for him, too. He was angry, irritable, and disgusted with himself for having allergies, and with the medical community for not having a superpill that would take care of his problem.

The program I outlined for him was similar to the one you are going to see shortly. It involved a dietary change and a complete nutritional supplement regimen. I told him two additional things, which I tell every patient. The first was that he needed to determine his triggers. This involved going through the list in chapter 2, and really trying to figure out if any of those allergens had relevance to his life. The second was to reduce or eliminate his exposure, no matter what. Much to my surprise, he embraced the cure wholeheartedly and has been drug-free for three years.

Medications

Many conventional allergy treatments are available. Antiallergy medications are some of the most commonly prescribed drugs in the world. They are marketed directly to the consumer in television and print ads, a practice I find deplorable.

Many of these drugs come with side effects that people find intolerable. The simplest method and probably the most effective way to avoid allergy symptoms is to stay away from the offending substance. Since that is close to impossible in its entirety, let's look at the mainstays of conventional medical allergy treatment: medications and allergy shots.

The types of medications used to treat allergies fall into these basic categories: oral antihistamines, nasal antihistamines, oral and nasal decongestants, nonsteroidal nasal sprays, steroidal nasal sprays, anticholinergics, and leukotriene modifiers.

Oral Antihistamines

These are the most common allergy medications and have been around since the 1930s. At best, they offer only temporary relief of mild allergy symptoms. These compounds work by blocking the products of histamine, the chemical that causes sneezing, nasal congestion, hives, and other allergic symptoms. These don't cure anything but do suppress symptoms. They are considered first-line therapy; however, antihistamines do not relieve nasal congestion.

The problem with most older antihistamines is their main side effect: drowsiness. Anyone who has to drive to work, or operate machinery, or perform tasks that require alertness has to avoid taking these medications or can only use them at night. In addition, they are very short-acting (four to eight hours, depending on the particular medication), so to be effective, they have to be taken several times throughout the day.

The older or first-generation oral antihistamines include diphen-hydramine (Benadryl) or chlorpheniramine (Chlor-Trimeton). These are the two most readily available that most people have used.

Other medications in this category include Atarax, Dimetapp, Peri-actin, Phenergan, Vistaril, and Tavist. The side effects of these drugs include drowsiness, dizziness, gastritis, dry mouth, tremor, urinary difficulties, loss of appetite, fatigue, depression, loss of sexual libido, nausea, and in some cases an increase in anxiety and nervousness.

Psychomotor impairment symptoms such as a decreased ability to concentrate and perform certain tasks can occur long after use of the drug has been stopped. The longer you take such drugs, the more likely these symptoms are to occur. These drugs also may leave you feeling hung over well into the next day.

Second-generation oral antihistamines include cetirizine (Zyrtec), fexofenadine (Allegra), desloratadine (Clarinex), and loratadine (Claritin). These drugs are much less likely to cause the psychomo-tor impairments described above, but they do have side effects. Two types of these medications were taken off the market soon after they were introduced—one because of an increased likelihood of causing seizures and death, and the other because of heart attacks and strokes.

Second-generation oral antihistamines are supposedly nonsedat-ing and nonexciting, although I have had patients report both. They need to be taken once or twice per day.

Nasal Antihistamines

These drugs are administered directly into the nose. According to the Joint Task Force on Practice Parameters in Allergy, Asthma, and Immunology, these should be considered as first-line treatment for people with allergies. The first drug of this kind is azelastine (Astelin), but it is currently not prescribed often. Another nasal antihistamine is in clinical trials.

Oral and Nasal Decongestants

These are effective in reducing nasal congestion but have minimal effects on sneezing or nasal secretions. Decongestants dry tissues in the nasal passages and reduce swelling in nasal membranes. They come in liquids, pills, sprays, and nose drops, both over-the-counter and prescription.

These drugs include pseudoephedrine, phenylephrine, and phenyl-propanolamine. Some of the more common trade names are Sudafed, Claritin-D, Deconsal II, Entex, and Triaminic.

Side effects include insomnia, loss of appetite, nervousness, and irritability. The side effects can be so bad that these drugs are not recommended for anyone with cardiac arrhythmia or high blood pressure. Phenylpropanolamine causes such a loss of appetite that it is popular in many over-the-counter (OTC) diet aids.

Nasal decongestants should not be used for more than two or three days in a row. Many people can get a rebound effect when they stop using these—their nasal congestion can be far worse than when they started. This condition is known as rhinitis medicamentosa. Don't abuse use of these sprays or you can become addicted to them.

Nonsteroidal Nasal Sprays

This category is dominated by cromolyn sodium. It can be used intranasally, inhaled, and even directly into the eyes. I believe this to be an extremely effective prophylactic agent for allergy symptoms. It is better at preventing symptoms than alleviating them. It is so safe that it has even been recommended for use by pregnant women—a recommendation that doesn't come easily.

Cromolyn sodium inhibits the release of histamine, must be started several weeks before your allergy season, and should be taken by anyone who has asthma or allergies, in my opinion. The only way to know whether this is going to work for you is to try it—its response rate is variable. Other nonsteroidal nasal sprays include nedocromil or Tilade, Nasalcrom, and Opticrom. Many of these are even available OTC.

Most nasal sprays work better if you use them after rinsing your nose with a saline solution. This rinsing removes the mucous secretions in the nasal passages and allows the medication to get directly to the lining of the nose. The rinsing also can remove any allergens such as pollen and dust mites that may be trapped by the mucus and causing a constant source of irritation. This can make an important difference to the effectiveness of these products.

Steroidal Nasal Sprays

These drugs work by reducing inflammation and opening the nasal passages so more air can be taken in through the nose. These drugs will inhibit the inflammatory pathways, immune system cells, and chemicals such as histamines, mast cells, basophils, eosinophils, leukotrienes, and cytokines. Nasal steroids indicated for the treatment of allergies include drugs such as beclomethasone (Beclovent), budenoside (Pulmicort), flunisolide (AeroBID), fluticasone (Advair Diskus/Flonase), mometasone (Nasonex), and triamcinolone acetonide (Nasacort).

Steroidal nasal sprays appear to be the most complete conventional treatment for allergies because they work against all the symptoms, including congestion, sneezing, itching, and nasal drippiness. However, there are many side effects.

Side Effects of Steroid Use

Many doctors downplay the significance of the side effects of long-term steroid use—in both spray and oral form—for allergies and asthma. They argue that these effects are a small price to pay for long-term control of allergies and asthma and alleviation of the symptoms. My argument is that since there are other ways by which people can learn to control their allergies and asthma, perhaps the price is too high. Only you as a patient and sufferer can make that decision. It is your right and duty to question your physician about these long-term risks. One study has indicated that even intermittent use of these drugs may increase the risk of death up to fivefold.

In patients using steroids, side effects will inevitably develop that should be monitored as closely as the allergies and the asthma themselves.

Some of the side effects are:

1. *Weight gain.* Your weight should be monitored monthly, and a proper exercise and diet program should be implemented at even the smallest weight gain.
2. *Glaucoma.* This condition can lead to blindness. You should have the intraocular pressure of your eyes measured at least annually.
3. *Cataracts.* This is a side effect that also can lead to blindness or decreased vision. Have your eyes examined at least annually.

4. *Hypertension.* Have your blood pressure monitored frequently, and don't let your doctor put you on a beta-blocker should you develop high blood pressure, as these types of drugs can precipitate asthma attacks.

5. *Glucose intolerance.* This can lead to diabetes, so it is critical to have your fasting blood glucose levels determined at least every three months, depending on the dose of medication you are taking, its frequency, your age and weight when starting steroid use, and family history.

6. *Peptic ulcer disease.* This is a frequent side effect of these medications. The symptom is usually heartburn but can be chest pain, stomach pain, or bowel disturbances. This can be effectively avoided by also taking the medication with food, antacids, or by also taking a drug such as Pepcid or Zantac.

7. *Myopathy.* This is a muscle disease that often leads to a wasting syndrome whereby you lose muscle mass.

8. *Mood disorders and insomnia.* Be on the lookout for abnormal mood swings; depression; or even symptoms of mania, such as decreased sleep or excessive spending of money.

9. *Hyperlipidemia.* This is an increase in your cholesterol level that may lead to heart disease or even stroke. Check your cholesterol level every six months to make sure this is not occurring.

10. *Osteoporosis.* In a study published in the *New England Journal of Medicine* in 2001, doctors measured the bone density of women age eighteen to forty-five who had asthma but no known conditions that caused bone loss and who were treated with inhaled steroids. Bone mineral density was measured at intervals of six months, a year, two years, and three years. They found a direct relation between a higher dose of inhaled steroids and small yearly decreases in hipbone density. This may lead to more hip fractures as a person with asthma ages. Since more and more people with allergies are being put on these medications, this will almost certainly be the case for those with allergies as well.

Some less serious side effects are worth mentioning. Inhaled steroids can cause hoarseness and yeast infections of the throat, which is candida or thrush; therefore, you should rinse your mouth and gargle after every inhalation. Don't swallow the water you gargle with. You must spit it out or you can develop a yeast infection in the rest of your GI tract that can be quite serious. Most physicians forget to tell their patients this simple but critical bit of information.

What about our children who take these drugs? Since there may be an adverse effect on bone growth and metabolism, and bone density also can be reduced, monitor your child's growth carefully.

Anticholinergics

The one drug in this class that has been approved for use by allergy sufferers is ipratopium bromide (Atrovent). It treats only the nasal dripping, not congestion, sneezing, or itching. Some people take this along with other medications if their nose runs constantly. This has a similar side effect profile to the drugs mentioned above.

Leukotriene Modifiers

These drugs were developed for treating asthma. Leukotrienes are ten thousand times more potent than histamines in causing an allergic response. Since allergies and asthma are so closely intertwined, scientists are looking at these drugs to treat allergies.

In several studies involving more than two thousand subjects, it was found that these drugs reduced symptoms in almost every participant and were better than a placebo in improving quality of life.

These drugs target the causes of inflammation rather than the symptoms associated with the inflammatory response, inhibit bronchoconstriction, and so far have an excellent safety record. The trade names of these drugs are Accolate, Singulair, and Zyflo. Side effects of these medications include headache, fatigue, fever, GI upset, cold/flu symptoms, thirst, and hives.

Allergy Shots or Allergen Immunotherapy

I wonder how many of you have been through these agonizing series of injections only to have your allergies remain and how many of you they have helped.

Allergy shots are also known as allergy desensitization techniques. These shots contain very small shots of the offending allergen. They are given a few days apart at the beginning of treatment and then monthly, and may last for years. A clinician is not able to predict who will benefit and who won't. They are usually very expensive and not always covered by medical insurance.

Clinical Uses

Allergy shots have been used since 1911. Since then, standardized extracts have been developed, optimal doses have been established, and schedules for the administration of these extracts have been determined. Despite these advances, this technique remains as much an art as a science.

Since many factors can affect the outcome of any course of allergy shot therapy, its effectiveness depends on how it is used, so I will explain how it should be used so you may determine whether the shots you have had or are currently receiving are being done properly.

Most studies show that allergy shots are effective for inhaled allergies. This holds true whether the person is being treated for allergic asthma or for allergic rhinoconjunctivitis (watery eyes, runny nose, etc.). The studies have shown them to be effective in allergy related to a variety of pollens, fungi (molds), dog and cat dander, dust mites, and cockroaches, when given *separately*. Allergy shots have not been shown to be effective for eczema, hives, food allergies, or stinging-insect sensitivity.

Allergen Extracts

These shots involve injection under your skin of extracts of the allergens you are sensitive to and that trigger your symptoms. The most commonly used extracts are derived from pollens of trees, grasses, and weeds, and from fungi, dog and cat dander, dust mites, and cockroaches. These are the most common allergen triggers for most people. I believe that most people, even those who don't suffer with allergies or asthma, when tested, will be allergic to at least one of the Big Five: dust, cats, molds, grasses, and pollen. These always seem to be positive, and most people receive shots for these five. Whether they help is another story.

The theory behind this treatment holds that the more of an extract that you are exposed to, the better the improvement in your clinical symptoms—up to a certain point. Increasing the dose after that holds no benefit. Allergy shots are best suited for those who have IgE-mediated sensitivity to allergens that cannot be avoided and that cause the allergic rhinitis and allergic asthma. Many people suffer from non-IgE-mediated sensitivities and allergies, and this treatment will not help them.

The shots themselves are usually given with a very small needle in the back part of the upper arm. The injection should be given slowly enough that you don't experience pain or swelling at the site. Also, pressure should be applied at the point of injection for up to a minute to prevent the extract from leaking. Dosages do not have to be reduced after a reaction at the site of injection. They should be reduced only if you had a full body reaction. Make sure they are given correctly.

The greatest risk associated with these shots is a systemic reaction that in some instances has proven fatal. Pregnant women, those on beta-blockers (any medication that ends in "olol"), and poorly controlled asthmatics are not candidates for this treatment.

Extract Selection

Allergy shots will work only for a specific allergen that is injected; therefore, you need a separate shot for everything to which you are allergic. This is more time-consuming, more laborious, more expensive, but more effective than giving them all in the same shot. The decision of what to include in your shot must be based on several factors:

- Knowledge of the offending airborne allergens where you live
- Patterns of allergen exposure
- Detailed clinical history focused on the relationship between your symptoms and exposure to the allergen

You must get the correct mix of ingredients and have them injected correctly; then you have a chance that this form of therapy will be successful. Otherwise, it is probably not worth the expense and the time. As with most other forms of allergy therapy, allergy shots work best when exposure to the offending allergen can be eliminated—in most cases, easier said than done.

How Allergy Shots Work

These shots should be given as early in childhood as possible because proper development of the immune responses should occur as early in one's development as possible. This most likely helps determine the progression of allergies.

It is believed that early administration of these shots can help to prevent becoming sensitized to certain allergens or can even help prevent the inflammation caused by exposure to the allergen and may therefore lead to a decreased incidence of asthma as well.

Make sure that you and your doctor are doing everything possible to ensure that this therapy does something for you. Make adjustments and monitor your progress. It may be helpful for you to keep a diary of symptoms and reactions so you can help your doctor plan accordingly. Don't expect him or her to make all the right decisions or to keep the best records. Take charge of your health and keep good records. Your doctor only sees you infrequently; you know your body and your symptoms, and the information you can bring to the table is invaluable.

Forming a Proper Program

As you can see, there are almost as many therapies for the treatment of allergies as there are allergens. The choices are vast, and none of them seems to be the definitive answer. While they may help to alleviate symptoms, most do little or nothing to help the underlying condition.

People with allergies tend to be allergic to many different things. That is why it is difficult to devise a proper treatment when the only thing you have to work with goes after symptoms and not the underlying issues. The cure you are about to undertake addresses the underlying issues that I feel cause the majority of allergy cases. I have been successful at alleviating the symptoms and decreasing the number and amount of medications that my patients use by having them follow the steps outlined in the program. This is your best chance of finding a cure because this program addresses the underlying causes of your body's hypersensitivity to so many things.

4

Conventional Therapies for the Treatment of Asthma

Pat, a forty-seven-year-old woman, came to see me because I had helped a friend of hers get off multiple asthma medications and she wanted to do the same. Pat was also pleased that I seemed to find out the reason why her friend was having so many attacks. She liked that approach and was wondering why none of her other doctors had ever inquired about this. I couldn't speak for them, of course, but what I can say is that in medical school, it is almost never taught to look for the underlying cause of asthma, just how to treat it with multiple medications.

I asked her to show me her medications. I was shocked. She was on the most medicines of any asthma patient I had ever seen. She took two different steroid medications; used three inhalers on an as-needed basis, which she admitted to using daily; two more inhalers, which she used on a regular schedule throughout the day; and several different allergy medications. She was most concerned about the steroid medications because as she entered menopause, she was aware that their use could leave her vulnerable to osteoporosis. While there certainly is a place for drugs in the treatment of asthma, we have come to rely too heavily on them and have not looked for the underlying reasons why people get these attacks.

I took a history of her allergen triggers and ran many blood tests, as well as other tests, including a food-sensitivity test, a candida blood test, and pulmonary function tests. Once the results came back and I started her on her program of dietary eliminations and changes, proper nutritional supplements, and a thorough cleansing of her environment, Pat began to feel better within the first week. By the end of three months, she was off three of her inhalers; and by the end of six months she was down to using only two of her medications on an as-needed basis only—which was rarely. Most importantly, she was not using either of the steroid medications. Three years later, she is free of her medications and breathing better than she ever has.

Official Guidelines

According to "Guidelines for the Diagnosis and Management of Asthma" of the National Institutes of Health (NIH), effective management of asthma relies on four integral components:

1. *Objective measures of lung function.* This is to assess the severity of a person's asthma and to monitor the effectiveness of treatment. This is done using pulmonary function tests.
2. *Pharmacologic therapy.* This involves the use of multiple medications. Until about 1992, asthma medications were prescribed only after wheezing began. Now, conventional medical doctors prescribe medications so that fewer attacks of wheezing occur; however, the death rate from asthma remains at about five thousand cases per year. What is all this medication doing?
3. *Environmental measures to control allergens and other airborne irritants.* This is effectively done through a thorough history to assess where changes can be made to reduce the allergen burden. This is often not done in the conventional model.
4. *Patient education.* In the conventional model, this is done simply to assess patients' compliance to their asthma treatment, not in teaching them how to be free of this disease. According to the NIH, effective management of asthma should have the following goals:

   - Maintain near-normal pulmonary function rates.
   - Maintain normal activity levels, including exercise.

- Prevent chronic and troublesome symptoms.
- Prevent recurrent flare-ups of asthma.
- Avoid adverse side effects from the asthma medications.

Conventional medical practice relies on medications for the majority of these outcomes. I believe that although drugs can be very useful, there is too much reliance on them and not enough focus on prevention, curing, environmental control, and patient education. If you look at the management objectives, they are simply that—managing a chronic disease. Isn't it time that we looked for a cure for this potentially deadly and certainly troublesome illness?

Do I Have Yeast/Candida?

Although there will be a complete review of candida shortly, I wanted you to take this little quiz to see exactly what I am talking about and to see if this is something that may be troubling you, too; I strongly suspect that it is.

William Crook, M.D., clearly formalized the important points to note in ascertaining the history of a patient with chronic candida. See if some of these points pertain to you. You are suffering from candida if you fall into one of these categories:

1. Have taken many courses of antibiotics
2. Bothered by fatigue, headache, or depression
3. Crave sweets
4. Often feel spaced out
5. Bothered by muscle aches and digestive problems
6. Unusually sensitive to tobacco, perfume, and other chemicals
7. Have or think you have food sensitivities
8. Have had jock itch, ringworm, athlete's foot, or nail fungal infection
9. Crave carbohydrates
10. Have sought help in vain from many different physicians

If you fall into any of these categories, chances are you have a chronic candida infection and should do something about it. Candida is something that must be addressed in every person who suffers from allergies or asthma.

Management—Step-by-Step

Determine your triggers. This is one of the most important things you can do to try to avoid further asthma attacks.

Reduce or eliminate exposure. Once you know your triggers, you need to do anything possible to eliminate them or at least reduce your exposure to them.

Watch for drug interactions. Aspirin, nonsteroidal anti-inflammatory drugs such as ibuprofen, and beta-blockers may lead to allergy and asthma attacks.

Exercise. This is important for keeping your weight down. We know that excess weight triggers increased asthma attacks. If you get an asthma attack while exercising, do something preventive before exercising, such as taking 2,000 mg of vitamin C.

Maintain proper pharmacologic therapy. Make sure you are on the right amount of medication to control your asthma with minimal risk of adverse side effects. I am constantly adjusting my patients' medications while they are improving. You need to be doing this as well, with the help of your physician.

Monitor your condition continuously. This must be done to ensure that you are on the proper medications. You may not need as much medication at certain times of the year; if your asthma is seasonal allergy-dependent, only take it during your bad season.

Treat the underlying condition. Have yourself evaluated for candida and food sensitivities. Eliminating them can make your asthma and allergies less troublesome.

See a specialist. See someone who is aware of the latest treatments and any complications that could arise.

Medications

There are essentially two different categories of asthma medications: anti-inflammatory, which help to reduce swelling in the airways; and bronchodilators, which are rescue medications used during an attack to relax the muscles around the airways and make it easier to breathe.

These medications are usually available in many forms, including inhaler, puffer, pill, or liquid.

Anti-Inflammatory Medications

These reduce inflammation within the air passages. For people with moderate to severe asthma, they are recommended for daily use. There are two types of these medications: nonsteroidal, and steroids or glucocorticoids.

Nonsteroidal Medications

For patients with mild disease, the cromones—cromolyn sodium and nedocromil—are excellent. I have found that these drugs are not used often enough. Many of my patients have never heard of them, and I place most of my asthma patients on them. They are relatively harmless, have few side effects, and should be considered in all cases of asthma.

The cromones inhibit allergen-induced airway narrowing as well as acute airway narrowing after exercise and after exposure to cold air and sulfur dioxide. They are not as effective as inhaled steroids for controlling inflammation or modulating airway remodeling, but they may be effective in preventing attacks and symptoms. This drug is named Intal or Gastrocrom and comes in a capsule, tablet, and powder form and even in a nebulizer.

Steroids or Glucocorticoids

The glucocorticoids can be subdivided into those taken orally and those inhaled. Oral steroids are prednisone, prednisolone, and medrol. They are often used in the treatment of severe acute asthma attacks. The use of these drugs has been shown to reduce emergency room visits and hospitalizations. Some patients who have severe asthma are kept on these drugs for extended periods of time, and the side effects can be severe.

Inhaled steroids are considered much safer, yet are not without risks. Use of the inhaled drugs provides symptomatic relief and can reduce airway hyperresponsiveness. The most popular drugs of this type are beclomethasone, triamcinolone, flunisolide, budenoside, and fluticasone. Some trade names are Azmacort, Aerobid, Beclovent, Flovent, Pulmicort, and Vanceril.

The many side effects associated with steroid use include cataract formation, osteoporosis, weight gain, and growth retardation in children. For a full explanation, please refer to chapter 3. While it is believed that these side effects are less pronounced in inhaled steroids, we just don't know for sure, so also try to avoid them if you can. Oral steroids have more side effects, but the inhaled versions are not harmless. Because some of these drugs are inhaled, the most commonly seen side effects are in the nose. These include nasal bleeding, nasal irritation, and nasal septal perforation. These are not harmless medications despite what your doctor may say.

Bronchodilators

These drugs act primarily to dilate the airways by relaxing the bronchial smooth muscle. Several different types of these drugs are available, including beta-adrenergic agonists, methylxanthines, and anticholinergics.

Beta-Adrenergic Agonists

These are considered the medication of choice for the treatment of acute flare-ups of asthma attacks and for the prevention of exercise-induced asthma attacks. Prolonged regular administration of these medications can have detrimental side effects. There is now some concern that there is a relationship between use of these drugs and dying from asthma. I therefore recommend they be used on an as-needed basis only, for acute airway obstruction.

The most frequently prescribed drugs of this type are albuterol, pirbuterol, metaproterenol, and the long-acting salmeterol. Trade names include Proventil, Alupent, Maxair, Serovent, Ventolin, Breathaire, Bronkometer, and Advair Diskus.

The most common side effects of this type of medication are gastric upset and excitability, nervousness, or agitation. This can be especially troublesome if the medication is taken at night or by school-age children. These can lead to poor school performance, decreased ability to concentrate, and marked decrease in appetite. Children on these medications may get diagnosed with attention-deficit disorder, when the reason is actually their medication.

Methylxanthines

The one you are most likely to be familiar with is theophylline; I used to take it when I was a child with asthma. This is a mild bronchodilator and is known as a phosphodiesterase inhibitor. A proper blood level must be maintained for this drug to be successful.

If there is too much in your bloodstream, you can begin to experience nausea and vomiting as the first warning sign. Seizures, disturbed behavior (especially in children), rapid heart rate, abnormal heart rhythm, difficulty urinating in older men, elevated blood sugar, and elevated potassium levels have been reported.

Theo-Dur, Slo-bid, Slo-Phyllin, Tedral, and Theolair contain theophylline.

A compound that is similar to a methylxanthine is caffeine. Therefore, anything with caffeine, including coffee, tea, soda, chocolate, and even decaffeinated beverages if they are not herbal teas, may make someone with asthma feel better if that person consumes one of these substances.

Anticholinergics

These are used infrequently in the treatment of asthma. The most common one is ipratropium or Atrovent.

Ephedrine

This is generally not as effective as the inhaled agents and thus is used less frequently. There are many natural preparations of this, called ephedra, on the market. It is also found in many Chinese herbal preparations and in homeopathic remedies for asthma. Ephedra has been around for many years to treat the symptoms of asthma, but because of the side effects, I never recommend it. Side effects include nervousness, irritability, excitability, and abnormal heartbeats.

Leukotriene Modifiers

These are the newest agents in the battle to control asthma symptoms. They have been with us only since 1996. Zafirlukast (Accolate) and montelukast (Singulair) are leukotriene receptor blockers. In the lungs they block the action of leukotrienes, which are ten thousand times more potent than histamines in causing an inflammatory response. The other drug in this class, zileuton (Zyflo), works slightly differently, by inhibiting the synthesis of leukotrienes released by the mast cells in the lungs.

While these drugs have been helping thousands with their symptoms, long-term safety studies in children are not yet available, although they should be soon. These drugs seem to be able to alleviate asthma symptoms, improve objective measures of airway function, and decrease the need of rescue medications and inhaled steroids, according to all the studies on the subject. Singulair also has been shown to reverse the bronchospasm brought on by exercise.

Over-the-Counter (OTC) Medications

Primatene Mist and Sudafed are very popular OTC preparations for asthma. Both contain ephedrine. Primatene tablets also contain theophylline. They should be used only as needed for an acute asthma attack. Other OTC bronchodilators include Bronitin Mist, Bronkaid Mist, and Medihaler-Epi. All contain the drug epinephrine bitartrate and must be monitored closely.

Cough Medications

Many people with asthma experience coughing as one of their primary symptoms. The two types of cough remedies are expectorants and cough suppressants. In people with asthma, there is usually an abundance of thick mucus in the breathing passages. Therefore make sure you are using an expectorant, not a cough suppressant. A cough suppressant can make your symptoms and condition worse.

What Is on the Horizon?

As is always the case in medicine, many avenues of research are being investigated to find the next breakthrough. Asthma is certainly no exception. The newer drugs attempt to look at the misguided immune system behind an attack and to aim more precisely at the target.

IgE Antagonists

This is the most promising of the new kids on the block, and probably the next to be available. They work by neutralizing IgE antibodies, which are normally produced whenever your body encounters something that shouldn't be there, such as a cold, flu, or allergen. IgE then causes the release of histamine, leukotrienes, and other chemicals, leading to an asthma attack. These new drugs will block the binding of the IgE to the mast cell and basophil, thus stopping the chain reaction.

Third-Generation B-Agonists

There are several of these being investigated that hopefully will not have the lethal side effects that the current ones do.

Cytokine Antagonists

These are in the first stages of human trials. Some of these antagonists target a chemical of the immune system called IL-4. Other research in this area is looking at the role of other immune system cells known as IL-12, Gamma-interferon, IL-10, and IL-18.

Others

Other treatments being studied include adhesion molecule antagonists, transcription factor antagonists, oligonucleotide, and other gene therapies. There is even a vaccine currently in development. Hopefully one or more of these will be the magic bullet that all asthma and allergy sufferers are looking for. Until then, you are going to have to be more aggressive in attempting to cure your disease yourself.

Finding a Cure

Conventional treatment of asthma is based on a patient's response to the drug therapy. Thus it creates a dependence on these drugs, and since the patient's symptoms are relieved, it causes most patients not to try to find a cure for their disease. Asthma patients can get very complacent when their medication is working successfully.

The medications are not successful at getting to the real cause of your allergies or asthma, and the long-term side effects can be horrendous. I want to give you a program that will get you out of my office and into the world, without adverse side effects.

Most of my patients have been immensely successful trying to get off their medications, breathing more easily, and leading a more normal life. This will be possible for you, too, if you follow the advice in this book. You can do something about your allergies or asthma; following the advice in this book is the first step toward a great recovery program.

PART II

Allergies and Asthma: A Complementary Medical Approach

5

Understanding Food Sensitivities: The Allergy and Asthma Cure Step One

Because this book is written for several different types of people, I want to set up a little road map to help you navigate through its next two parts. At the end of this and the following seven chapters, I list the steps you need to take the cure properly. There is a lot of information you must know, so this map will make it easier to understand. It will help if you make notes.

If you are:

1. Overweight with allergies, follow steps 1 to 7.
2. Nonoverweight with allergies, follow steps 1 to 4, 6, and 7.
3. Overweight with asthma, follow steps 1 to 6 and 8.
4. Nonoverweight with asthma, follow steps 1 to 4, 6, and 7.

If you are reading this book because you suffer from any of the other inflammatory or allergic conditions such as eczema, psoriasis, or hives, please follow the appropriate allergy pathway.

Asthma, Allergies, and Fatigue

Helen, a twenty-seven-year-old woman, came to see me because she had asthma that was triggered by her allergies. When asked, she also reported general symptoms of fatigue; inability to concentrate, mostly in the afternoons; bloating; and occasional headaches. However, her main concern was her asthma. She was on three different medications, and her symptoms were getting worse. I was her last resort. She had been to several allergists and had taken every available test. She was skeptical about our visit because she really didn't see what else I could do that might make her well. She was in my office only because her friend had recommended me so highly.

I took a detailed history to find out what her allergen triggers might be, and to discover what else might be wrong with her. I explained to her that I was going to take some blood tests and physically examine her. Immediately she said she had all the tests done and didn't want any more. She brought me several years of records and asked if they would be sufficient.

While I could certainly appreciate her frustration, no doctor can begin treatment of a patient without first conducting his or her own investigation into the cause or causes of the problem. I told her that I did not want to retest her for the allergies, but I did want to do some blood work that she had probably never had done before—tests for food sensitivities and a test for candida. She then asked if I had read her reports—she had the RAST tests for foods and wasn't allergic to anything. How would my tests be different?

This is a phenomenon I experience in my office from time to time. Most allergy and asthma patients *have* been tested a lot. I don't blame them for not wanting to go through another exercise that may prove just as useless as all the others. The frustration level is high, and I don't want to add to that, but a food sensitivity test is essential to the program that I am about to describe, and more likely than not, you have never had one. Therefore, let me tell you what I told Helen, but in more detail.

Food Sensitivities vs. Food Allergies

Food allergies can be life-threatening and must be monitored closely. Food sensitivities are not life-threatening, but they can be troublesome and, in my opinion, are an underlying cause of asthma, allergic rhinitis, eczema, hives, and even acne.

Unlike an allergy, a food sensitivity or intolerance is an adverse reaction that does not necessarily involve the immune system. We are unsure as to the exact mechanism. Lactose intolerance is one such example. This does not involve the immune system per se, but the person lacks the enzyme that digests milk sugar, or lactose. A person with this or a different type of food intolerance can experience such symptoms as diarrhea or stomach pain after consuming the offending food. I believe that the majority of people who think they are lactose-intolerant are not. I have never had a patient who was unable to resume eating milk products again after taking this cure—even if the person had previously been lactose-intolerant.

People can be sensitive to food additives, too. This group can include artificial or natural colorings, flavorings, sweeteners, preservatives, or any of the multitudes of chemicals that have entered our food supply and that we ingest regularly. Up to 70 percent of all Americans think they are sensitive to one food or another, but statistics show that only 1 to 2 percent of adults actually suffer from food allergies. That is still three million people. An estimated 6 to 8 percent of children under age three also have an allergy to food. Except for rare instances, and for the most deadly, such as peanuts, nuts, and seafood, most children will outgrow their allergies by the time they are ten years old. Twenty percent of parents believe that their child has a food allergy.

While the figures for true food allergies are most likely correct, food sensitivities may be affecting the remaining 70 percent of adults and the rest of the 20 percent of our children who think they have problems with certain foods. These people are being ignored by the traditional medical community, who believe that food sensitivities don't exist. If this is true, then food sensitivities may be the most underdiagnosed medical problem in American history.

Do I Have a Food Sensitivity?

I suspect that you have some food sensitivities; most people do. Usually the foods we crave the most are the ones we are most sensitive to. Please take this short quiz to see if food sensitivities can be a problem for you.

Do you suffer from:

SYMPTOM	YES/NO
Irritability	_____
Difficulty breathing	_____
Rashes	_____
Difficulty losing weight	_____
Anxiety	_____
Asthma	_____
Hives	_____
Acne	_____
Mental dullness	_____
Inability to concentrate	_____
Hunger all the time	_____
Panic attacks	_____
Forgetfulness	_____
Headaches	_____
Wheezing	_____
Eczema	_____
Weight gain	_____
Binge eating	_____
Confusion	_____
Hyperactivity	_____
Sinus trouble	_____
Dizziness	_____
Itchy eyes	_____
Ringing in the ears	_____
Stuffy nose	_____
Sore throat	_____
Palpitations	_____
Vomiting	_____
Abdominal fullness	_____
Arthritis	_____
Being easily frustrated	_____
Insomnia	_____
Watery eyes	_____
Itchy ears	_____
Mucus drainage	_____
Cough	_____
Irregular heartbeat	_____

Diarrhea   _____
Muscle weakness   _____
Swollen hands or feet   _____
Difficulty learning   _____
Drowsiness after meals   _____
Dark circles under the eyes   _____
Runny nose   _____
Postnasal drip   _____
Throat tickle   _____
Nausea   _____
Constipation   _____
Chronic fatigue   _____
Short attention span   _____
Poor work habits   _____

Scoring:

If you answered yes:

0–4: I don't know why you are reading this book. Give it to a friend or loved one.

5–10: Food sensitivities are contributing to your not feeling well; get the test done.

11–20: You must address this issue of food sensitivities or you will never feel 100 percent again. Run and get the test done.

21–51: I am so glad you bought this book and are about to start on this program—it is going to change your life.

Although this list is broad, I am trying to get you to see that there are many symptoms that *may* be related to food sensitivities. We consume food several times each day. Given the complexity of the food chain, it is conceivable that we are sensitive to something along the way. Most of the foods that we eat are not pure, whole foods, so even if it is not the food itself, it is highly probable that we are sensitive to something that gets placed in our food supply somewhere between the farm and the dinner plate.

Since many of the symptoms that I have listed above are minor, most people do not see a cause and effect with the food they eat. In some instances it may be harder to find the offending food than to suffer the symptoms. My patients are always amazed when I point out that so many of their minor symptoms may be related to what they are eating. Once they eliminate the offending foods and feel so much better, they are again amazed that something as simple and as basic as food can cause so many problems for them.

As humans, we grow accustomed to minor irritations all the time—smoke, traffic, our boss's voice—that we forget that life can exist without these things and that we would probably feel better for it. Think how much better we feel on vacation; but, a week after we are back, most of us forget we ever went. Most of us have lived with food sensitivities for so long that we are used to feeling the way we do. It is important to rid our bodies of this low level of inflammation that we tolerate every day. An inflammatory process on this constant a level may indeed be the basis for our problems with allergies and asthma. Once this inflammation is gone, we can start living our lives feeling well again—and eliminating our allergies and asthma along the way.

Testing for Food Sensitivities

There is a big controversy, even among complementary medical practitioners, over the proper way to test for food sensitivities, because of a lack of data on many of the testing modalities. I am going to tell you about the different ways to test and the one I have found to be most effective.

The two major ways of testing for food sensitivities are blood tests and elimination diet techniques. Neither is definitive. There are several minor ways of testing for food allergies, too, which I consider less scientific; but there have been practitioners who have successfully used these techniques for many years so I will briefly mention those as well. They are electrodermal screening, muscle testing, and pulse tests.

Blood Tests

There are several different tests on the market that attempt to isolate your food sensitivities utilizing your blood. This is the way I evaluate food sensitivities in my practice. There are several different types of these tests that you should be aware of.

RAST

These tests were previously described in detail. They are highly vari-able from lab to lab, meaning that the results are hard to duplicate. They measure only IgE reactions. IgE tests are good at looking at true food allergies but not food sensitivities, because food sensitivities are usually not IgE-related. Therefore I do not recommend these tests.

Cytotoxic Test

This is the test that I previously preferred. In my first book, *Feed Your Kids Well,* I discuss this test in some detail. It is not readily available, and technicians trained to administer it are in rare supply, so don't look for it in your local doctor's office. This tests your white blood cells against a number of food products. The biggest criticism of this test is that it uses food that has not been predigested because stan-dardized predigested food products are unavailable. Therefore, many think this is an inaccurate portrayal of what you may be truly sensi-tive to. I do not recommend this test at this time.

Histamine Release Test

This blood test measures the histamine released from your white blood cells when they come into contact with a particular food extract. The problem is that it is uncertain whether this release of his-tamine would correspond to an adverse reaction you would get if you ate the particular food. I do not use this test in my practice.

ALCAT Test

Although I hesitate to mention company names, I feel I must in this situation because it is the test I use most frequently. It is available from AMTL Corporation, and you can find their contact information in chapter 15, "A Resource Guide." It has been in use since 1986, and it works quite differently from any of the other tests I have previously described.

In this test, your blood is incubated with the individual allergens in separate little containers—each for a different food. More of your blood is then incubated with the diluent—the liquid the allergens are held in. This ensures that any reaction your blood shows is from the food and not from the liquid it comes in. This is important because each person's blood is then measured against his or her own control or baseline, not a standardized control, which is a potential source of error.

Your blood is then incubated for $1\frac{1}{2}$ hours longer. Thirty minutes of this is at body temperature so that immune system reactions can begin to take place. The rest of the time is at room temperature so that your blood and its immune system components will stabilize before going through the next step.

Your blood and its own control will then pass through a channelizer, where a reagent is added to each little container. This causes the red blood cells to be destroyed; only the white blood cells, where all the reactions take place, remain.

The reactions this test measures are multifaceted. Things other than ordinary IgE are looked at. Complement or C3 and C4, IgG, IgA, and IgM are all measured. These are different components of the immune system that may all lead to inflammation and hence allergies and asthma. That is the main reason why I think this test is important. Since we really don't know the true mechanism of food sensitivities, anything that can be measured, probably should.

Once the red blood cells are destroyed, the channelizer records these different components using a coulter counter technique. This technique uses the principle of electrical fields to count the number of cells and the size of the cells that are different from your own standard or control. Although various parameters are measured, the test is easily reported to the physician and the patient in an easily understandable way.

The Food Sensitivity Awareness Program

Your food sensitivities are reported as negative, 1+, 2+, or MPOS. Regardless of the brand of test you will eventually take, you will more than likely get a reading like the one I am describing. When the results of the test are available, I advise all of my adult patients to avoid the foods marked 2+ or higher. If you get the official readout from an ALCAT test, these foods are marked in orange and red. For all of my patients under the age of 14, I recommend that they avoid any food that isn't negative.

The foods for which you test positive should be avoided for three months if you stick to your diet perfectly and eliminate the offending foods, and for three to six months if you are less than perfect. You do not have to eliminate the foods forever—just until your body has had time to heal and for the inflammation to be reduced. Three to six months may seem like a long time, but the inflammatory process in your body took a long time to develop and needs some time to heal. Be patient and you will get the same great results as my patients.

While you are going through this process, it is important to remember to rotate the foods you are eating—don't eat the same foods all the time. Often, when people try new things, once they get it right, they don't want to change for fear of doing something wrong. In this instance, this could be troublesome because you don't want to develop new food sensitivities. That could happen if you eat the same foods repeatedly. I know this can be trying at times, but the results will speak for themselves.

The test I usually order consists of the hundred most common foods that people eat. Your doctor—if he or she is using this cure—can order additional foods if you eat something regularly that is not on the list of tested foods, but I have found the hundred to be the most cost-effective.

The other tests that look at food sensitivities are from companies such as Great Smokies and Doctor's Data. They are very reliable companies, and you may be able to find a doctor to administer one of these tests even if they won't administer the ALCAT. These tests are all relatively expensive, and sometimes insurance companies will not pay for them. I have found them to be invaluable resources in helping my patients overcome their allergies and asthma and breathe better, and they are generally worth every penny.

Drawbacks of Food Sensitivity Blood Testing

The biggest drawbacks to these tests have always been in their reproducibility. Food sensitivities are not food allergies. The exact mechanisms by which food sensitivities affect the body are not completely understood. A food allergy will cause the same reaction every time you encounter the offending food. This will not happen with a sensitivity because the reactions are much more subtle and do not work through the IgE mechanism of allergy. I don't consider a particular test to have failed because it is not 100 percent reproducible. No blood test is completely reproducible. But your symptomatic improvement will speak volumes for the importance of these tests.

The problem with food sensitivities is that they usually are a silent process in the body. The reactions they cause may take place in areas of the body where you do not experience pain or discomfort like in your tissues or organs. This chronic immune assault can take place at each meal until your immune system is overwhelmed. You might then find yourself going from doctor to doctor trying to find answers and not addressing the real culprit; you may not even have realized that the culprit existed. That is why the recovery process may take so long.

Food sensitivities often produce delayed reactions. Most people know if they are allergic to a particular food. The reaction can be life-threatening and serious. With food sensitivities it can take days, months, or even years to become problematic; therefore, it is not always easy to see the cause-and-effect aspect of food sensitivities.

Food sensitivities are complex reactions that occur through a combination of factors that are not completely understood. Food sensitivities may be related to how much of a given food you ingest, how frequently you ingest it, what form you ingest it in, what else you are eating with it, and many more factors. Our eating habits are diverse, and we don't eat the same way all the time, nor do we eat the same combinations of foods. It is difficult to standardize for all the variables when it comes to the foods we eat. That's okay; be assured that they exist.

Although food sensitivity testing is not an exact science, I feel that if your doctor has a certain level of expertise and is comfortable with a certain technique, you can greatly benefit. By taking my cure, you will be benefiting from my years of using the exact technique with my patients that I am describing to you.

General Elimination Diet Technique

If you do not have a doctor who, or a convenient lab that, can do any of the tests I mentioned, or if you are an ultrapurist or simply can't afford one, then you must go through the process of an elimination diet. You do not have to do this if you have had one of the blood tests. Doing this is not as easy as a simple blood test. If you are going to embark on my cure you need to narrow your list of potential food sensitivities and must do it one way or another. I have seen too many successes by eliminating them to have any doubt that this is a real phenomenon.

A general elimination diet will exclude groups of foods, several at a time. This should be followed by a specific elimination technique to further pinpoint your food sensitivity.

Since this is going to take some time, I recommend that you start with the most common food offenders, which include: dairy, wheat, and corn. The next two biggest offenders are chocolate and foods containing salicylates. The latter is especially helpful to eliminate if you or your child has any attention deficit or other behavioral issues. This doesn't seem like an extensive list, but wait until you see everything in which these foods are contained. If you already suspect a particular food, you should eliminate it as well, especially if it falls into one of these categories.

Each category of food must be eliminated for three weeks. When following an elimination diet, there can be no deviation—not even once, because of the delayed timing of many food sensitivities. Medications you normally take should be continued, but try to avoid all others. I especially think you should try to eliminate any allergy medication you are taking, as this may cloud the results. The basic plan is this: (1) Choose a category and eliminate those foods for three weeks; (2) keep a symptom questionnaire; and (3) do the specific elimination technique for the foods that bother you. Then it is on to the next category, and the process is repeated until you have gone through the Big Five.

Dairy Elimination

This category includes cow's milk, goat's milk, sheep's milk and any cheese made from those ingredients. It also includes dried, evaporated, or skim milk. Cheeses of any kind as well as any foods that may contain cheese, butter, ghee, or margarine are also in this category. Also, ice cream, sherbet, creamed soups, puddings, some gravies, and any food product that may contain whey and nondiary milk substitutes that contain any casein, since this is a milk protein. Some nonmilk cheeses, like some soy cheeses, also contain casein, so check the ingredients list. Calcium supplements also may be included in this category if the calcium source is from milk or one of its proteins. Protein powdered drink mixes and protein energy bars all most likely contain one of these forms of protein, so check the ingredients list carefully.

Eggs are allowable in this grouping, as are all meats, vegetables, and fruits during this stage of the elimination process.

Wheat Elimination

In this category eliminate all of the grains, whether they contain gluten or not. The gluten-containing grains are barley, buckwheat, oats, rye, and wheat. The nongluten grains are millet, rice, wheat bran, oat bran, spelt, teff, amaranth, quinoa, and wild rice.

Wheat is in an enormous number of foods. This category also includes breads, cookies, cakes, crackers, pretzels, wheat germ, wheat starch, pasta, graham crackers, pastry, pies, bread crumbs, waffle batter, pancake batter, ice cream cones, malted milk, beer, sauces, soups, and any food containing noodles. Also, you may want to eliminate the following foods unless you can be sure you have made them at home and they contain no fillers: sausages, hamburgers, meat loaf, potato croquettes, fish cakes and fish sticks, fish rolled in crackers, chili, and canned baked beans. Also avoid any food that may be breaded, such as chicken fingers, chicken or veal cutlets, Wiener schnitzel, and the like. This category also contains such vegetarian staples as breaded tofu and seitan.

In addition, the following foods must be avoided during this phase of your elimination diet: cocomalt, gin or any grain-based alcohol, Ovaltine, Postum, whiskey, biscuits, popovers, rolls, most cereals, lima bean flour, doughnuts, frozen pies, dumplings, zwieback, bouillon cubes, chocolate candy, matzos, mayonnaise, most prepared meats, liverwurst, and bologna. These lists are not meant to be exhaustive, but just to give you an idea of the foods you must avoid in each category.

Foods you may eat during this phase of your elimination diet include most meats, vegetables, soy flour, and fruits.

Corn Elimination

Corn is almost more common than wheat, and it may be harder to do this set of eliminations than any of the others. Many processed foods contain corn, and many of our drinks are sweetened with high-fructose corn syrup. Cornstarch, corn oil, and cornmeal also must be avoided, so please check labels thoroughly. Since corn has become so widely used in our food processing industry, we are seeing more and more people sensitive to it.

The obvious foods to avoid are the cereals made from corn, as well as fresh, frozen, roasted, and canned corn. Grits are made from corn, as is popcorn. Many medications and vitamins contain corn as a filler, binder, or even sweetener. Corn is in nonfood items as well and should be avoided as much as possible during the trial elimination. These include adhesives, aspirin, paper cups, paper cartons (such as for milk or orange juice), gelatin capsules, gum on envelopes, stickers, stamps, tapes or labels, spray starch, bath and body powders, throat lozenges, plastic food wrappers, some toothpastes, and even paper plates.

Other foods to avoid include brandy, bacon, baking mixes, beer, breads, candy, ketchup, most cereals, cookies, fried foods, baking powders, batters for fish, chicken, or meat, beets, bourbon, pastries, carbonated beverages, cheeses, chili, Chinese food, instant coffee, vinegar, powdered sugar, pasta, sausages, thickened soups, peanut butter, cream soups, pickles, leavening agents, yeast, chewing gum, baby food, margarine, gelatin desserts, corn chips, gin, bologna, frankfurters, grape juice, cured ham, jams, jellies, sherbets, canned peas, cream pies, salad dressings, canned vegetables, tortillas, and most sauces.

I have not even mentioned everything that may contain corn. Corn is ubiquitous in our society and is an extremely difficult category to eliminate. However, if you are going to do this correctly, you should eliminate everything you can that has corn or one of its derivatives in it. The safest foods that you can eat while attempting to eliminate foods in this category include all meats, vegetables, and fruits.

Chocolate and Caffeine Elimination

This seems relatively easy at least where the foods are concerned, yet there are many hidden foods in this category, too. You must also eliminate any food that contains cocoa, cocoa butter, cola drinks (including diet sodas), and carob. Also exclude tannic acid teas, coffee, and any other caffeinated beverages. The obvious foods here include chocolate candy, cake, ice cream, chocolate milk, and anything that is chocolate-flavored or -coated. In addition, some dark rye breads and other dark breads may contain cocoa or chocolate.

This is probably the easiest category of foods to try to eliminate and you may want to start in this category, as there are many other foods that you can eat while attempting to do this elimination.

Salicylate Elimination

Probably the most common thing you could name from this group is aspirin. However, many preservatives, artificial flavorings, coloring agents, and other various chemicals and foods are in this category, but this information is not on the food labels. The words to look for on food labels are calcium-disodium EDTA, BHA, sodium sulfite, sodium lauryl sulfate, and monosodium glutamate— all are additives that are also salicylates. Salicylates may be found on a food label under the name acetylsalicylic acid (aspirin).

Fruits that contain salicylates and that should be eliminated are almonds, apples, apricots, blackberries, cherries, cucumbers, pickles, currants, grapes, raisins, nectarines, oranges, peaches, plums, prunes, raspberries, strawberries, and tomatoes.

An example of other foods that most likely contain some form of salicylates are margarine, breakfast cereals, jams, jellies, lunch meats, toothpaste, mint flavors, gelatin products, candy, cake mixes, bakery products, frankfurters, and mint flavorings, including wintergreen.

An example of drinks that may include salicylates or additives are apple cider, apple cider vinegar, red or white wine, red or white wine vinegar, soft drinks, diet drinks, tea, beer, Kool-Aid-type products, gin, and most distilled beverages except vodka.

Any medicine that contains aspirin and there are many of these, including some throat lozenges, perfumes, mouthwash, and anything containing artificial color, artificial flavorings, or preservatives, are all in this category. There are too many to list here, but one of the most common artificial colors is tartrazine.

This is an extremely broad list but one whose elimination I have seen to be very effective for certain groups of people. In some children and adults, elimination of these foods can help in concentration, attention deficit disorder, and other behavioral problems. The Feingold Institute has popularized this program as a treatment for these very common issues.

The foods that can be eaten when attempting to eliminate in this category include any meats that have nothing artificial in them: fish, except those processed or prebreaded; eggs; milk and milk products; any fruit I have not mentioned in this category; acetaminophen-based pain relievers; and most vegetables.

Specific Elimination Diet Technique

If you follow the technique just described, it will take fifteen weeks to determine which categories of food may be giving you problems. To reiterate, this is something I have never asked a patient to go through; I use the blood tests.

After using the general elimination diet technique, to find the specific food, you must start reintroducing foods into your diet systematically: Add a specific food to your diet for five consecutive days in larger quantities than you would normally consume, while eliminating everything else in that category. Test first for foods in which you have a particular interest or are most suspicious of and eat most often.

Specific Elimination Diet Technique Worksheet

You must keep a worksheet as you undergo this long process. A way to keep track of these particular reactions is to reintroduce a new food, then write down the name of the food and whether you notice a reaction, don't notice a reaction, or can't tell if you have a reaction.

If you do not have a reaction in the five days and have been eating the food in larger quantities, then it is believed that this food is not an offender for you. By the time you have finished reintroducing the foods in each category, you should have a good handle on which foods you are sensitive to. You should be able to compile a list that you can use to begin the rest of the program.

Other Complementary Approaches

I would like to mention a few more common ways of testing for food sensitivities that you may have come across.

Pulse Testing

This test has a long history and has been used for many years with apparently good results. Essentially, it measures your heart rate before and after exposure to a particular food. It is easy to take your pulse, and the easiest place to measure it is on your wrist. Face your palm upward; then place two fingers on the outside of your wrist (the thumb side) and you should easily be able to find your pulse. The pulse should be strong and steady in this location.

To test the response to a certain food, eat a single food at a time— preferably one you suspect—and look for any change from the way your pulse normally feels. Your pulse may become quicker, or can even slow down and become weaker. You also may feel an irregular beat if the food is an offender. Because food sensitivities can often induce a delayed reaction, this test has limitations; I do not use it.

Muscle Response Testing

This technique is also known as applied kinesiology. It simply means that the relative strength of your muscles is used to uncover allergies, sensitivities, or other misalignments in the body.

It is believed that this technique uncovers blockages in the electro-magnetic energy fields when your body is exposed to an allergen, and is based on the premise that a strong muscle supposedly becomes weak when it becomes exposed to an allergen. The usual approach is to place the suspected allergen in your hand and then test certain muscles. You lie down, and the person administering the test pushes against your arm muscle while you resist. If you are holding in your hand something you are sensitive or allergic to, the arm muscle will become weak and you will be unable to resist having it pushed down. Supposedly, this technique can detect even hidden sensitivities in some patients, according to its proponents.

Generally I am very skeptical about the accuracy of this technique. However, I have seen some practitioners perform it and be very accurate in their assessment of the patient's food sensitivities. If you go to a practitioner who is very gifted and has been doing this technique for a long time, you will probably get good results. If not, then this test probably will not be very accurate for you. I do not do it in my own practice.

Electronic Testing

These are electronic devices that attempt to do the same thing that muscle testing does, only with more technology involved. Some of these machines are EDS (electrodermal screening) and EAV (electroacupuncture device). The machines were designed to verify the relationship between acupuncture points and their corresponding organs. They do this by measuring electric current (remember, our bodies are electrical machines) at particular acupuncture points by reading the galvanic skin response. This technique has been used to measure food, chemical, dental, and many other types of sensitivities. The test involves your holding a metal probe in one hand while another metal probe is placed at various acupuncture points throughout your body. The electrical response is measured at these points and stored in a computer attached to the machine. The electromagnetic energies of the various allergens are already in the machine, so it is possible to test for a wide variety of offending substances. I do not use this test in my practice.

If you have one of the ailments discussed in this book, I am certain that you have food sensitivities, and you must figure out what they are so you can proceed with the cure. Just as allergies and asthma go hand in hand and one can't be explained without the other, so it is with candida, food sensitivities, and a condition called leaky gut. The next chapter will tie all these together for you.

Please review and follow the following simple checklist to make sure you have gotten to the bottom of your food sensitivities.

The Allergy and Asthma
Cure Step One: Review

1. Have a food allergy test done; in my practice, I usually recommend the ALCAT test.
2. Have your physician order the hundred-item test. If you follow an atypical diet or think that your sensitivities may be related to additives, dyes, or certain foods that are not part of the hundred most common foods, then add those foods to the test

individually. If you suspect additives, there are separate panels
for those; test for them as well.

3. When you get the results: adults, eliminate any food marked
   2+ or MPOS and that is red or orange on the final printout.
4. When you get the results: children under fourteen years, eliminate any foods marked 1+, 2+, or MPOS. Those foods are
   correspondingly in the yellow, orange, or red boxes.
5. If you get a different blood test done: for children, the same
   rule applies—any food that is not negative should be avoided;
   for adults, any food 2+ or higher should be eliminated.
6. Eliminate the offending foods for three months if you eliminate the food and follow your diet perfectly.
7. Eliminate the offending foods for up to six months if you are
   less than perfect with your eliminations.
8. Try not to eat the same foods every day; you'll possibly
   develop new food sensitivities.
9. If the food is in the negative category, don't assume it can be
   eaten. Always defer to the diet chapters.
10. Keep a symptom questionnaire.
11. *If no blood testing is available,* or if you wish to be a purist,
    follow the general elimination diet technique first, with an
    emphasis on the following categories of foods: dairy, wheat,
    corn, chocolate and caffeine, and salicylates—one at a time.
12. Eliminate one category of food at a time for three weeks with-
    out cheating once.
13. Keep a symptom questionnaire and compare it at the begin-
    ning of the three weeks to the end of the elimination period. If
    there is a positive sign, then proceed to 14. If not, then pro-
    ceed directly to 15.
14. Follow the specific elimination diet technique for that particu-
    lar category of foods.
15. Follow the general elimination diet technique for the next
    major food category.
16. Repeat 12 to 14 until each category has been eliminated and
    you have your list of specific food sensitivities.
17. Save this information as you read farther.
18. Read about candida and its relationship to leaky gut; then be
    prepared to take the cure.

6

Understanding Candida and Yeast: The Allergy and Asthma Cure Step Two

Mary, a sixty-one-year-old female, came to my office because she was interested in getting off her allergy and asthma medications. Her asthma started when she was menopausal and was slowly getting worse each year. After taking a thorough history, I also uncovered that she had a chronic sinus infection. Upon asking, she couldn't remember the last time that her sinuses were clear. She almost never breathed through her nose anymore and thought it was all related to her allergies and asthma. Her sinus condition, which consisted of a runny and stuffed nose and headaches from time to time, seemed to be worse in the spring and the fall. She was often on antibiotics and was forty pounds overweight.

I performed several tests for her that included food sensitivity, routine chemistry and hematology tests, and a candida test. She had heard of all the others, but did not know what a candida test was. She reluctantly agreed to have it done. It was positive, and she was highly sensitive to yeast on her food sensitivity test as well.

This did not surprise me because many people who have asthma and allergies also suffer from chronic sinus problems and, in my experience, have issues with candida. If you are looking for the underlying reason why you have difficulty breathing, have the candida test done because it is probably going to be positive.

As I explained to Mary, most sinus infections are caused by fungal infections. Candida is a fungus. Antibiotics are commonly given to treat sinus infections, yet antibiotics do not treat fungal infections. In fact, they cause the fungi to overgrow in our bodies. The overuse and overprescription of antibiotics have made candida a common occurrence.

Upon hearing this, Mary was shocked. She had been given at least ten courses of antibiotics in the past three years and had diligently taken each of them. Now she was mad and vowed to finally get to the bottom of her allergies and asthma. I outlined her program, and her allergies, asthma, and sinus problems cleared up in three months. She has not needed to use any of her inhalers or any allergy medication and certainly no antibiotics for the past three years. She is thrilled.

A Fungus among Us

Each of us has candida in our bodies. It is supposed to be there. It makes up part of what we call the normal flora of the body.

Candida is just one form of yeast, or fungus, and *Candida albicans* is probably the most prevalent in and on our bodies. There are more than 250 species of yeast—they are found in almost every baked good, and we eat them all the time, like mushrooms. But more than 150 of these species of organisms are harmless parasites in our bodies. *Candida albicans* is a single-cell fungus and normally lives in the gastrointestinal tract, the mouth, and the vagina. The gastrointestinal tract is one of the largest components of the human body and is comprised of the esophagus, stomach, and small and large intestines. Candida also resides in the genitourinary tract, which consists of the kidneys, ureter, and urethra.

Candida is only a problem for us when it overgrows. Candida lacks chlorophyll and is not able to produce its own food; therefore, it acts like a parasite in the body. This is kept under control by friendly bacteria that also live in the body. Some of the ones you may be familiar with are lactobacillus, bifidus, and even *E. coli*. These organisms make up another important component of our normal flora. The lactobacillus bacteria make enzymes that help to fight an overgrowth of any undesirable bacteria. They help to keep our bowel tract in good shape and help to keep our bowels moving appropriately. The friendly or good bacteria use the yeast as their food. This relationship helps to maintain the balance between good and bad bacteria in our gastrointestinal tract. As long as there are enough good bacteria around, there should never be a problem.

However, that is not always the case. I have found candida to be a serious problem in most people with asthma and those who suffer with allergies. Understanding this yeast and its many consequences, and most importantly, how to eliminate this from our bodies is a cornerstone of my asthma and allergy cure.

Leaky Gut

Carol was a fifty-four-year-old female who came to see me because she wanted to be free of her asthma. I had helped one of her friends, and she didn't see why she still needed to be taking her three inhalers, since her friend no longer needed them. She had asthma since the birth of her second child about twenty years ago, and each year she seemed to be more and more allergic to things. Now she needed to use her inhalers daily.

I did my usual blood tests, which, of course, included a food sensitivity test. The number of foods she was sensitive to was unbelievable. Carol was thrilled because at last a doctor had found something wrong with her that could be corrected. She knew something was going on in her body, but no other doctor had told her what. I next explained to her that many people with food sensitivities have something called a leaky gut, which is usually related to candida and our GI tract.

A Healthy Gastrointestinal Tract

The gastrointestinal tract runs the length of our body from the mouth to the anus and covers literally miles of roadway. This is where all the nutrients to sustain life are absorbed by our bodies. If there is a breakdown anywhere along this system, it is safe to assume that we are not getting the nourishment we need to live a healthy life. This system is commonly known as the gut.

Since our gut is so important to our nourishment, it stands to reason that if it were healthy and functioning properly, then the rest of us ought to be, too. An unhealthy gut has been implicated in food sensitivities, chronic fatigue, fibromyalgia, irritable bowel syndrome, brain fog, eczema, hives, psoriasis, Crohn's disease, and ulcerative colitis, and I am now implicating it in allergies and asthma.

A healthy gut allows properly digested food to pass into the bloodstream so it may be used for fuel. It also acts as a barrier to keep out foreign invaders such as bacteria, viruses, and undigested food particles.

In simple terms, picture your intestine; it is made up of cells. These cells form a barrier against disease while allowing nutrients to pass through. Imagine that these cells are held together very closely, like a honeycomb. That is similar to what a healthy gut should look like.

An Unhealthy Gastrointestinal Tract = Food Sensitivities

Now imagine that this honeycomb begins to fall apart or allows gaps to form between individual cells. There are now holes between cells that shouldn't be there; thus the protective barrier they provided begins to break down. Keep in mind that this is all on a cellular level.

Once this barrier is broken down, poorly digested food particles and bacteria can flood our system. These are not supposed to be there, so they act as antigens, and our immune system will do what it is designed to do: it triggers an antibody response. These antibodies will cause a cytokine release, which then activates our basophils and eosinophils, causing irritation and inflammation that is not necessarily confined to our digestive tract. These antibodies circulate throughout our body, and that is why food sensitivities can cause systemwide reactions. These are the same reactions that occur whenever our bodies come into contact with any other invader or allergen—hence the connection to allergies and asthma.

Now that you have built up antibodies to certain foods—usually the ones you eat most often because that is what is leaking into your gut—your body will become sensitized to those foods. Therefore, the minute you eat those things again, your body immediately recognizes them as foreign, and the inflammatory reaction takes place more quickly. If the goal of any treatment for allergy or asthma is to reduce inflammation, then inflammation must be reduced everywhere it can be. Since we eat at least three times per day, this is a potentially huge source of inflammation that must be eliminated.

Now that you understand how your gut can actually become leaky, the next part of this puzzle to understand is that candida is lining every part of our digestive tract. Once these cells have openings between them, the candida can then travel to other parts of your body and take up residence in places where they like to grow—warm, moist, membranous regions such as your lungs and sinuses. Since the candida is not supposed to be there, it will cause inflammation and discomfort—stuffy nose, sinus headaches, difficulty breathing, wheezing, and even muscle aches.

Symptoms of a Leaky Gut

Most of the symptoms associated with a leaky gut are systemic, since candida produces toxins that can circulate throughout our bodies. These symptoms include abdominal pain, bloating, gas, fuzzy thinking, diarrhea, constipation, memory or concentration difficulty, fatigue, malaise, indigestion, mood swings, hypoglycemia, breathlessness, itchiness, stuffed nose, runny nose, sinus problems, nervousness, palpitations, and many more. I know that these symptoms sound vague, and they may be related to something else, but if you are suffering from allergies or asthma, chances are you have some of these other symptoms and never knew they were all related—and all related to candida.

How Do I Know if I Have a Leaky Gut?

The diagnosis is made through symptoms and history. If you have the above symptoms and all other causes have been ruled out, then most likely you have a leaky gut. The biggest indicator I use is if the person has more than ten food sensitivities. If he or she has fewer than ten, but more than five and has many of the symptoms I have described, then I assume that a leaky gut is present. There is usually no other explanation for the patient's feeling the way he or she does. If a patient of mine has allergies or asthma, I always treat for a leaky gut.

I do not do any special testing to determine if a leaky gut is present, but some practitioners will perform an intestinal permeability test. This involves drinking a solution of two sugars named lactulose and mannitol. Mannitol should easily pass through the gut whether it is healthy or not and get readily absorbed. Our guts are impermeable to lactulose, so it should be very difficult to have this pass through our intestine and get absorbed by the body. Therefore, the test measures your urine and looks at the ratios of the two sugars to see if your gut is leaky. If there is a high percentage of the lactulose in your urine, it is considered diagnostic for a leaky gut. This test is readily available throughout the country; you can find out where to get it done in chapter 15, "A Resource Guide" in the Complementary Medical Information section.

Candidiasis

This is the medical term used to describe the overgrowth of candida. There are several reasons why this overgrows. The most common cause is the overuse of antibiotics. This can mean using antibiotics too often, or for too long a time. The antibiotics will kill the good bacteria in our digestive tract, along with any of the harmful bacteria we may be taking the antibiotics for, but not the candida since candida is a fungus and antibiotics do not kill fungus, giving it room to grow.

I am sure that most of the women reading this book can relate to this scenario because when women take antibiotics, quite often they will get a vaginal yeast infection. The same thing happens in your intestinal tract and may very well be the cause of your allergies and asthma.

Most Americans get yeast infections from overusing antibiotics. If you have used antibiotics repeatedly and/or more than once in a three-month period, you probably have a yeast infection. Besides, most upper respiratory infections, ear infections, and sinus infections—the most common reasons why patients take antibiotics—will resolve on their own without any medication, because they are most often caused by a virus or a fungus—two things not treated by antibiotics.

In a study published in 1994 in the *Journal of Allergy and Clinical Immunology*, researchers from the University of Virginia found that oral antifungal medication such as ketoconazole and fluconazole helped a number of patients suffering from asthma. It would therefore stand to reason that there must be a fungal component to this illness because that is what these two drugs kill.

Other Causes of Yeast Overgrowth and Leaky Gut

Overuse of antibiotics is the main but not the only reason for this outbreak of candida and leaky gut. The most common causes other than antibiotics are hormonal imbalances; steroid medications; other medications, including nonsteroidal anti-inflammatory drugs; environmental toxins and chemicals; viruses; chronic stress; gastric or duodenal ulcers; Crohn's disease; ulcerative colitis; overuse of alcoholic beverages; and my favorite, diet.

Hormonal Imbalances

Hormones, such as progesterone and birth control pills, as well as pregnancy also can lead to candidiasis. These are the main reasons why there tend to be more yeast infections in women than in men. Progesterone rather than estrogen is the culprit and hence PMS may be related to an overgrowth of yeast and why pregnancy can lead to candidiasis.

Steroid Medications

Basically anything that suppresses the immune system can cause an overgrowth of candida and a yeast infection. Steroid medications are a big cause of immune suppression. The medications in this category include prednisone, prednisolone, beclomethasone, and many other inhaled steroids that people with allergies and asthma use daily. People with allergies and asthma are prime candidates for yeast infections because of their habitual use of steroid medications. Others who also use steroid medications frequently for their illnesses include those with Crohn's disease, lupus, and arthritis. They, too, are at risk for developing a case of chronic candidiasis and leaky gut—not only because of their use of these medications, but also ulcerative colitis, Crohn's disease, and ulcers cause damage to the integrity of the lining of the GI tract and lead, once again, to an overgrowth of candida, and multiple food sensitivities.

Other Medications

Other medications that can lead to an overgrowth of candida include chemotherapy or radiation therapy, because these treatments will suppress the immune system; any drug that can cause inflammation in the gut or stomach such as aspirin; and nonsteroidal anti-inflammatory drugs such as Tylenol and Motrin. These drugs can cause stomach ulcers and irritation of the lining of the GI tract and can therefore lead to candida overgrowth, food sensitivities, and a leaky gut. These are some of the most commonly used over-the-counter drugs in the world, so please be aware of these side effects. Antacid medications that are usually given to avoid the GI upset when you take these types of medications can in themselves lead to candida because they can increase the pH of the stomach high enough for the yeast to overgrow. Your normal stomach pH is about 2 or 3; candida thrives in an environment of about 4 to 5, and antacids may increase your stomach pH to that level.

Environmental Toxins and Chemicals

Anything that can suppress the immune system can lead to an overgrowth of yeast. This group includes pesticides and herbicides (from the residue on the food you eat), motor vehicle exhaust, lead, arsenic (commonly found in tuna), mercury, and other heavy metals. People who work in these industries commonly have candida, but due to our polluted environment, we should all be aware of these causes.

Miscellaneous Sources

This is another group of very common disorders that could lead to candida and leaky gut. They include recurrent Epstein-Barr virus or cytomegalovirus, chronic fatigue, recurring colds or flus, and major surgery.

Chronic Stress

When we suffer from chronic stress our bodies produce less secretory IgA—one of our first lines of defense and a necessary component of a healthy gut. This lines the digestive tract and helps to keep those cells tightly glued together. With less being produced, your body is more prone to candida and leaky gut and thus food sensitivities. Stress is a powerful suppressor of the immune system, and it is important that we learn to control this in some way. It may not always be easy, but we have to try.

Diet

I firmly believe that the standard American diet (SAD) is the real culprit behind most chronic yeast infections. While all of the other things I have mentioned may lead to a yeast issue, diet is what completely fuels the reaction and heats it up. A forest fire will die without oxygen, and an overgrowth of yeast will die without sugar. The SAD is overrun with sugar.

Overconsumption of sugar is bad for many reasons. One is that since candida cannot manufacture its own food, it will utilize sugar as its fuel of choice. Another reason why sugar leads to an overgrowth of candida and a leaky gut is related to the immune system. I have mentioned how any damage to the immune system can lead to a yeast overgrowth. Sugar is a major contributor to a damaged immune system. In fact, a teaspoon of sugar can suppress your immune system by 56 percent; 2 teaspoons, by 78 percent. There are more than 2 teaspoons of sugar in a glass of orange juice or a candy bar, and the average person consumes 33 tablespoons every day, or 158 pounds per person per year.

I think diet is the most important part of the cure you are about to undertake. Actually, diet is one of the most important steps to good health that any of us can take. It is the cornerstone of being healthy and must be corrected before anything else.

Symptoms of a Yeast Problem

In all my years of treating people with allergies and asthma, I have come across only one who did not test positive for candida.

There are many symptoms of yeast—probably many things that you are currently experiencing. Some of the more common symptoms are bloating, gas or flatulence, eructation (burping), indigestion, heartburn, asthma, hives, runny nose, stuffy nose, sinus headaches, clogged sinuses, fatigue, acne, eczema, and earaches.

Some of the more common symptoms in women of childbearing age include recurrent vaginal infections, PMS, recurrent urinary tract infections, sexual dysfunction, painful intercourse, endometriosis, uterine fibroids, sugar cravings, and infertility.

Some of the more common symptoms in men include fatigue, headache, digestive symptoms such as I described above, muscle and joint pain, depression, food sensitivities, sugar craving, memory loss, and possibly sexual dysfunction.

In young children, some of the more common symptoms are crankiness, constant colds, excessive diaper rash, sleep problems, ear infections, problems with attention span, and hyperactivity.

In older children, some of the more common symptoms are irritability (hard to tell in a teenager), fatigue, a "spaced out" feeling, poor school performance, headaches, and even depression.

Another important symptom that may affect all age and sex groups and that is extremely common is brain fog. I know that doesn't sound like a medical diagnosis, but I think that many of you have it. This refers to a detached state of mind, poor concentration, memory difficulties, forgetting why you went into a room, and difficulty making routine decisions, such as how to get to a store that you have gone to each week for twenty years. Things just don't seem to be coming to you as quickly as they once did. This can be the most debilitating and annoying yeast symptom for many people.

I do not mean to say that all of these symptoms, many of which are relatively minor, are always attributable to yeast. There could be some serious medical reasons why you suffer from some of these symptoms. But if you and your doctor have ruled out any major difficulty, then you must think of yeast as the culprit and do something to get rid of it or the symptoms and the yeast condition will only get worse. Don't let your doctor tell you that all your symptoms are in your head. Yeast may be the culprit.

In my experience, yeast is a huge contributor to the problems that those with allergies and asthma have. I have helped so many people with allergies and asthma improve dramatically once yeast is eliminated from their bodies that I wish more doctors wouldn't ignore this syndrome because it wasn't taught in medical school.

Candida Questionnaire

In *The Yeast Connection* by William Crook, M.D., Dr. Crook devised a checklist to help patients determine if the symptoms they are suffering from are connected to a yeast problem. I have revised the checklist so it is a little easier for me and my patients to use. His questionnaire is divided into three sections. The first asks about your medical history, the second focuses on yeast-related symptoms, and the third focuses on more minor symptoms of a chronic yeast problem. I combined them all into one, and pared it down significantly to the following thirty questions:

QUESTION	YES/NO
1. Have you taken antibiotics four or more times in one year?	_____
2. Have you been bothered by recurrent prostatitis or vaginitis?	_____
3. Do you sometimes feel spaced out?	_____
4. Do you feel sick yet are found to be normal at your doctor visit?	_____
5. Have you used steroid medications of any kind?	_____
6. Are your symptoms worse on moldy, damp, or muggy days?	_____
7. Do you crave sugar or carbohydrates?	_____
8. Have you had any fungal infections, such as athlete's foot?	_____
9. Do you experience headaches?	_____
10. Are you depressed?	_____
11. Do you suffer from abdominal bloating?	_____
12. Do you suffer from flatulence or gas?	_____
13. Do you move your bowels once per day or more?	_____
14. Do you suffer from PMS?	_____
15. Do you have hypothyroidism?	_____
16. Do you suffer from headaches?	_____
17. Do you have asthma?	_____
18. Do you have seasonal allergies?	_____
19. Are you more irritable than usual?	_____
20. Do you suffer from eczema?	_____
21. Do you suffer from chronic hives?	_____
22. Do you suffer from insomnia?	_____
23. Do you suffer from bad breath?	_____
24. Do you suffer from postnasal drip?	_____
25. Do you suffer from sinus problems?	_____

26. Do you suffer from recurrent colds? _____
27. Do you suffer from recurrent earaches? _____
28. Do you have difficulty concentrating? _____
29. Do you suffer from hypoglycemia? _____
30. Are you moody? _____

Scoring:

If you answered yes:

0–5: You do not have a chronic yeast infection and should skip the rest of this book; give the book to a friend.

6–10: You have a mild case of chronic candidiasis and need to start a yeast-free diet. Your allergies and asthma will almost definitely improve on this program.

11–20: You have a moderate case of chronic yeast and need to be treated with antifungal nutritional supplements and be on a yeast-free diet. Your allergies and asthma will definitely improve with this program.

21–30: Many people, especially those reading this book, fall into this category. Allergy and asthma sufferers need to eliminate yeast so they may begin to breathe freely again. The diet and nutritional supplement program in this book will help you breathe easier and possibly get you to throw away some of those nasty medications.

Blood Tests

Available blood tests are not the most perfect way to diagnose a yeast infection because they are unreliable. Most conventional doctors may refuse to give you the tests or may never have heard of them. However, they are readily available at most major labs. A negative finding doesn't mean that you don't have a yeast problem. History is more important than any blood test in diagnosing candida.

Candida Antibody Test

This is the test I administer most frequently in my office and the one offered by most labs; it measures the level of antibodies your immune system has made to fight the candida. The test I administer measures the IgA, IgM, and the IgG antibodies. These are important distinctions because they enable me to determine if the infection is new or old. Since our bodies face candida daily, there is usually some underlying level of candida antibody present, even in someone without symptoms. This test is far from perfect, but coupled with the results of your quiz, can give you a good indication if yeast is causing your allergies and asthma.

Candida Antigen Titer Test

This test measures if there are any yeast antigens or toxins in your blood. The test is not reliable because it gives a lot of false negatives. It is not a test I administer.

Cultures

This is a test that I never administer to help determine if a patient has a yeast problem. I mention it simply because there are many practitioners who do administer it. Many body parts and fluids, such as urine, as well as nasal, throat, and vaginal secretions, can be cultured for yeast, but this test usually looks for candida in the stool. Because candida can be present normally in our bowel tract, yeast can be detected in someone who is normal. More importantly, one should look for the level of the beneficial lactobacilli in a stool culture if you are going to bother to have a test of this type done. If the lactobacilli level is low, then the yeast has a good chance to overgrow.

Food Sensitivity Tests

These tests can show whether you are sensitive to brewer's or baker's yeast. Brewer's yeast is in fermented alcohol such as beer. Baker's yeast is in the baked goods that many of us love so dearly.

There are many ways to diagnose an overgrowth of yeast/candida in your body. Many of them are controversial. Just because something may be controversial doesn't mean there is no merit to it. If your conventional medical doctor tells you that you couldn't possibly have candida and your symptom checklist is full, then you definitely have it, even if your blood test is negative and your doctor doesn't believe it exists. Sometimes in medicine you have to think outside the box. If scientists didn't do just that, we would be in serious trouble. Unfortunately, most physicians no longer think, they react; and, therein the problem lies.

Allergy and asthma patients are unique in that what works for one may not work for another and what sets one off has no effect on another. While that is certainly true, one constant I have seen in my practice is the preponderance of yeast and yeast-related symptoms in people with allergies and asthma. The other constant is that they get better when they are on a program that eliminates this problem. Who could ask for more?

Where Do I Go from Here?

Repairing a leaky gut, getting rid of candida, and coming to terms with your food sensitivities are the key components of the allergy and asthma cure. These three are so interconnected that you can't discuss one without discussing the other two. Candida causes a leaky gut, which leads to food sensitivities. Food insensitivities can cause a stomach imbalance, which could lead to an overgrowth of candida, which can lead to a leaky gut. No matter which comes first, the results are the same—increased levels of inflammation and many systemic consequences, including allergies and asthma.

We are now set to embark on the rest of the treatment program. Each of the three big culprits needs to be treated. The treatment can be done simultaneously and is essentially the same for my allergy and asthma patients. The results are going to amaze you.

The Allergy and Asthma
Cure Step Two: Review

1. Fill out the candida questionnaire.
2. If you answered yes to more than five questions, assume you have a yeast condition.
3. Get a confirmatory blood test (candida antibody) if possible.
4. Follow the yeast-free diet in chapter 8.
5. If you want to lose weight, combine the diet in chapter 8 with the diet in chapter 9. I will explain how to do this.
6. If you don't want or don't need to lose weight, then just follow the diet in chapter 8.
7. Follow the dietary recommendations for three months if they are followed perfectly.
8. Follow the dietary recommendations for six months if followed less than perfectly.
9. Read chapter 7 (step three) next.

PART III

The Allergy and Asthma Cure Nutritional Program

7

Setting the Stage: The Allergy and Asthma Cure Step Three

Now you have all the information you need to know if you are getting treated correctly. And you have all the information you need to find out what is truly causing your allergies or asthma. Since there are so many important aspects to taking this cure, I want to make sure that you are really ready to go to this next step.

Many patients can feel overwhelmed at the start of any new program. That is only natural. I am sure you have been to many physicians and have begun to lose all faith that they are ever going to make you better. The program you are about to begin has been proven in my patients, their relatives, and their friends. There are several important steps to review before we go to the next, most important, healing phase of the program. Please follow this next set of steps to keep you on the road to recovery.

Allergen and Asthma Trigger List

This is the list of the most common triggers for people with allergies or asthma that spur on attacks. I want you to think about these triggers long and hard and not just rush through them. If you are unsure about whether these things bother you, then answer yes. It is better to err on the side of caution in this situation.

Please respond yes or no to each of the following questions:

DO YOU THINK YOU ARE
SENSITIVE TO OR HAVE YOU HAD A REACTION TO: YES/NO

Aerosol sprays _____
Air pollution _____
Animal dander _____
Aspirin or ibuprofen _____
Cockroaches _____
Cold outdoor temperatures _____
Dust mites _____
Estrogen _____
Exercise _____
Foods _____
Gastroesophageal reflux disease or heartburn _____
Heredity _____
Molds (both indoor and outdoor) _____
Obesity _____
Perfumes and other chemicals _____
Pollens _____
Respiratory infections _____
Sinus infections _____
Smoke _____
Strong emotions _____
Sulfites (preservatives in red wine, beer,
dehydrated soups, salads, and other foods) _____
Thunderstorms _____
Viruses _____

There are probably more things you answered yes to than you had thought. When you put all these things in one place, it is amazing how they all seem to add up. Maybe you are starting to believe you can do something about your allergies and asthma after all. Now that you have this bit of information, begin to remove as many of these things from your life as you can. Some may be impossible, but follow the tips in chapter 2 for some suggestions. Let's try to make this work.

Symptom Questionnaire and Worksheet

This worksheet will help you see how well you are doing on the program, and help to keep you motivated. It will also come in handy when trying to put things back into your diet. The steps I have outlined and the ones you are about to do are designed to help heal your body from the constant assaults of daily life. We have been under so much assault for so long that we have forgotten how to feel any differently or any better. This program is not about treating your symptoms only, although you will become less symptomatic. It is about decreasing the inflammation that is the underlying cause of your problems. That is a far cry from just using all the drugs you have taken through all the years you have suffered and leaving it at that. The allergy and asthma cure is going to help you live your life the way it was meant to be lived. The simple cost of all that is just following the program.

Respond to each question, even if the symptom does not pertain to you now. I have found that most allergy and asthma sufferers have a particular set of problems that are their "normal" symptoms; but since you would be following the program for several months, there may be symptoms that only occur from time to time. If there is a symptom that usually bothers you but isn't on the day you take the quiz, answer it the way that symptom usually makes you feel.

Rate each symptom on a scale of how troublesome it is to you, with 1 being not troubling and 10 the most troubling—it bothers you every day. When you give each symptom a number, you will be able to see how much better you are feeling on the cure. I have left room for you to include symptoms not on the list.

There is also room on the questionnaire for you to list medications you are taking. I am sure that once you start the program, you are going to need less and less medication, so track these as well. If you are going to participate in this program and reduce your medication, please discuss this with your personal physician first.

SYMPTOM	START	WK. 2	WK. 4	WK. 6	WK. 8	WK. 10	WK. 12
Shortness of breath	—	—	—	—	—	—	—
Wheezing	—	—	—	—	—	—	—
Coughing	—	—	—	—	—	—	—
Runny nose	—	—	—	—	—	—	—
Postnasal drip	—	—	—	—	—	—	—
Chest tightness	—	—	—	—	—	—	—
Disrupted sleep	—	—	—	—	—	—	—
Stuffy head	—	—	—	—	—	—	—
Stuffy nose	—	—	—	—	—	—	—
Watery eyes	—	—	—	—	—	—	—
Congested head	—	—	—	—	—	—	—
Congested ears	—	—	—	—	—	—	—
Itchy eyes	—	—	—	—	—	—	—
Itchy ears	—	—	—	—	—	—	—
Sore throat	—	—	—	—	—	—	—
Fatigue	—	—	—	—	—	—	—
Other symptoms	—	—	—	—	—	—	—
Medication	—	—	—	—	—	—	—

This questionnaire applies to the first healing phase of the cure. Make a clean copy of it so you can continue to follow your symptom progression through the breathing-better phase as well. This may be the first time you have taken a systematic look at a disease that significantly affects your quality of life. The possibility is there for you to allow your body to heal and for you to feel better. Let's make that happen, but you need to help.

The Allergy and Asthma Cure
Step Three: Review

1. Review the allergen and asthma trigger list.
2. From the triggers that you checked off, ensure that you are doing or have done everything I suggested or that you can think of to remove these things from your environment or diet.
3. Have a food sensitivity test.
4. If you can't have a food sensitivity test, follow the general elimination diet technique as outlined.
5. List your food sensitivities and allergies so you can make sure those foods are eliminated when we discuss diet.
6. Fill out the symptoms questionnaire and keep it handy.

8

The Healing-Phase Diet:
The Allergy and Asthma
Cure Step Four

In my practice, I see many patients who need to lose weight. Living and being healthy—including losing those unneeded pounds—should be things we do without great effort. Unfortunately, this is a seemingly impossible goal for most of us in this society, which is just not set up for us to have a healthy body. We are bombarded with wrong messages in the media and are encouraged to live in an unhealthy way regarding food. We are bombarded by advertisements for the wrong foods. In addition, we are encouraged by our peers to eat incorrectly; for example, at parties, at work, even when out to dinner, we are tempted to eat the wrong things, even when people know we are on a diet or a special food plan. Yet these same people would never think of offering an alcoholic "just a small one." Also, we tend to think that maybe we can eat a little of what we want, "just this once." Again, if we were alcoholic and had quit, we would never think that way. We have to change our mind-set about food and get the rest of the world to go along with us. The proverbial deck is stacked against us and we have to try to change—if not the rest of the world, then perhaps just for ourselves and those around us.

Food is the basis of life. There is no truer adage than "you are what you eat." If anyone wants to be healthy, then he or she must have the correct diet, the cornerstone of good health. Everything else is additional. The term "nutritional supplement" says it all. Those pills should supplement what we are eating, not be our nutritional basis while we continue our same eating habits. Everyone is always looking for the Holy Grail or one magic bullet. There is none, and as disappointing as this may be, we must get used to that and do what is necessary to ensure our good health.

A proper nutritional plan is going to take some work and dedication, and the first step on your road to recovery is having the courage to do this and to get motivated and stay that way. You have to believe that you can do this and be committed to it—as if your life depended on it. There can be no excuses for not following the program, because you are the one who is going to benefit. I know you can do this, and for those of my patients who follow this to the end—and that is most of them—they are still grateful to this day for the opportunity to breathe better and be rid of their medications. Many of my patients initially felt that they could not do the cure. They thought it would be too hard. Once they started seeing the results, most of them stuck with it. For perhaps the first time in your life, take control of your asthma by taking control of your diet. If nothing else, this is probably the only thing you haven't tried and it is definitely worth the shot.

Read This First

To simplify the program so you can better follow it at home, I am going to give all of the dietary recommendations in two chapters for the healing phase of your program—one for weight loss and one for those who don't need or want to lose weight. A separate chapter will then be provided to help you learn how to transition your diet from the strict healing phase to the breathing-better phase.

This chapter presents the yeast-free healing diet for those who don't need to lose weight. Chapter 9 will teach you how to incorporate this yeast-free program with a weight-loss program. For any reader who is overweight, whether you are interested in losing or not, I recommend that you follow the weight-loss guidelines. You may as well. As long as you are doing this program anyway, why not lose weight in the process?

If you think that this recommendation is just for vanity, let me assure you that it is not. There have been several studies linking dietary habits to asthma. Most of these studies were done on children, but the data certainly can be extrapolated to include adults. In one study, at the University of Sydney in Australia, it was shown that the consumption of dietary sugar was a contributing factor to the development of asthma. They recorded the dietary habits of 213 children and measured their ability to breathe normally while exercising. The children (102) whose airways were hypersensitive to exercise ate 23 percent more sugar than those who didn't. This is especially important because asthma is often exercise-induced in many people. It was for me when I was a child, sixty pounds overweight and unable to breathe.

Another recent study, published in the medical journal *Thorax*, looked at the dietary intake of essential minerals and vitamins that have an antioxidant component. The study showed very strong evidence that nutrient-depleted diets, such as the standard American diet (SAD), caused an increase in asthma. Changes in diet absolutely influence how well you breathe—despite what your conventional medical doctor may tell you. This is why I am a very strong proponent of getting the diet in top shape first and then adding other necessary changes with it.

Standard American Diet (SAD)

This is a great acronym for the way most Americans eat because it truly is sad. It's worse than that—it's pathetic. More than 80 percent of all adults over age 25 and 33 percent of all children in the United States have a weight problem. Too much sugar, carbohydrates, and fats, not just one or the other, is consumed. People in the U.S. consume 158 pounds of sugar per year per person. This roughly translates to 33 tablespoons every day. Sugar suppresses our immune system, and candida loves to eat sugar; this can't be good for anyone who suffers from allergies or for the person with asthma.

Carbohydrates are the new villains of overweight people. I agree with this in general but not to the extent that most other low-carbohydrate diet doctors profess. There must be some carbohydrates in our diet. However, there are good carbohydrates and ones that are not so healthy for us. Most of us eat the ones that are not so healthy for us, such as white pasta, white bread, and pretzels, to name a few.

Fats have been so vilified in our society that many of us have forgotten how important they can be for proper nutrition and health. The reason fats got such a bad name is because of the type of fats we consume. As a rule, we tend to eat the unhealthy fats—polyunsaturated ones. We also eat too many foods that contain transfatty acids or partially hydrogenated oils.

People with asthma need to pay particular attention to fats because good fats are anti-inflammatory. Omega-3 fatty acids have an anti-inflammatory effect, while omega-6 fatty acids promote inflammation. Yet we eat an abundance of omega-6 fatty acids every day. Omega-6 fatty acids are the ones that you see in most every processed food, and they are known as transfats or partially hydrogenated oils. The most common oil that we all think is healthy is canola oil. It is exceptionally healthy when cold and one of the most unhealthy when heated. If you get nothing else out of this book, don't ever cook with canola oil again. I recommend you use olive oil, or even better, macadamia nut oil. The two are similar in quality, but macadamia nut oil has a healthier profile. It is the highest in monounsaturated fats, making it the heart-healthiest oil. It has the lowest amount of omega-6 fatty acids, and it has one of the highest smoke points—greater than 400°F. The smoke point of olive oil is only 200°F; therefore, macadamia nut oil is the perfect oil for cooking, as it is very difficult for this oil to turn rancid. Not only that, it also has a light, nutty taste, which makes it great for dishes where you would not want to use a heavy olive oil. I believe so strongly in this oil that I have begun to recommend to my patients that they take a tablespoon of it every day by itself, just like flaxseed oil, to reap all the health benefits they can. Good examples of omega-3 fatty acids are those in fish.

To put it simply, anyone, but especially a person with allergies or asthma, needs to increase his or her intake of omega-3 or omega-9 fatty acids, and severely limit the omega-6 fatty acids. Increasing your intake of macadamia nut oil, olive oil, fish, and nuts, while decreasing the amount of canola oil, other oils, and processed food of any kind, including baked goods, can only make you healthier.

I will briefly mention saturated fats. Everyone thinks these are terrible for you. Most are, but some are quite healthy and can be found only in red meat. Conjugated linolenic acid (CLA) is one example. It has been shown to be cancer-protective and is being widely used to help people lose weight as a nutritional supplement.

Getting Started: The Healing Phase

The first place to start in the allergy and asthma cure is to control the amount of yeast in your diet. This is the first ruling principle, and since this has a direct correlation on food sensitivities and leaky gut, you will be helping to control those issues, too. Nutritional supplements will be beneficial in helping you do this and will be discussed shortly.

This phase of the diet should last about three months. That is the same for everyone, whether you want to lose weight or not. This phase allows your body to heal from all the inflammation it has received from all the assaults placed on it every day. If you want to lose weight, and it takes longer than three months, then you would stay on the weight loss part of the diet until you reach your desired weight. The restrictions from this healing phase would be lifted. I will explain how to combine the two in chapter 9, on weight loss.

Bear in mind, however, that the healing phase is a slow process and may take longer than three months. If you stray, then expect this phase to last about six months. If you follow this phase properly, you will probably begin to feel better almost immediately or at least within the first week.

However, you may feel worse in the first few days as your body learns to live without sugar and yeast, and as the stored toxins are eliminated. This is a perfectly natural response, and happens because the yeast is dying. As this occurs, your sugar cravings can be intense, and you may become nauseous, or even get diarrhea. Some patients have even had their skin break out. This does not happen to everyone, but it may. Either way, just stay with the program.

The object of this process is to restore your body's balance of bacterial flora. The yeast has overgrown your digestive system, and now we have to fix that imbalance. The first step is to eliminate sugar from your diet. This may sound easy or dreadful depending on your perspective, but it is very difficult considering the amount of sugar in almost everything we consume. It is even in things we normally wouldn't think of as having sugar, so I think it is important to do a quick review.

Sugar in All Its Forms

When we think of sugar, our thoughts naturally go to the usual suspects: candy, cake, ice cream, cookies, puddings, soda, doughnuts, pies, etc. These need to be eliminated from your diet.

Now you have to learn the hard part: the many disguises of sugar. When you read a food label, look for anything that ends in -ose or -ol. Other hidden sugars include honey, concentrated fruit juice, barley malt, brown sugar, cane sugar, high-fructose corn syrup, corn syrup, dextrin, molasses, hydrogenated starch, polyols, galactose, invert sugar, sorbitol, sorghum, mannitol, turbinado sugar, xylitol, maple syrup, rice syrup, cane sugar, fructose, and sucrose. Just because a food label says "no sugar added" doesn't mean the food is sugar-free. That simply means there is no additional cane sugar added, but they could have added any number of other ingredients and still legally put those words on the label. Food labels are regulated by the government, and because of that, manufacturers continually look for loopholes in the law that will entice you to buy the product without fully understanding the ingredients list.

Be particularly suspect of any food labeled as low-fat. When they remove the fat, they have to add something else so it will taste good; what they add is sugar. For example, fat-free Twinkies have more sugar than regular Twinkies, and both have an enormous amount of sugar to begin with. Another great hoax is low-fat baked potato chips. They may not have any fat, but they usually contain high-fructose corn syrup and dextrose, two forms of sugar. The best advice I can give is not to eat any prepackaged food. Look for the marketing buzzwords "low-fat," "no-fat," "no sugar added." If you see these, do not buy the product.

Sugar is in canned foods such as tomato sauce and baked beans; boxed foods such as rice pilaf mix, crackers, and stuffing; meats such as frankfurters, luncheon meats, fresh pork sausage links, and hams; and condiments such as pickles, prepared mustard, tartar sauce, and ketchup. In fact, most brands of ketchup contain more sugar than ice cream does.

To make matters worse, there are more than three hundred standardized foods that may contain sugar without having to mention it on the label. These include salad dressings, canned vegetables, peanut butter, vanilla extract, and even iodized salt.

Is Fruit Just a Well-Disguised Sugar?

The answer to this question is a resounding yes. If you were thinking that you didn't eat any sugar, but consume a lot of fruit, you are not in any better shape. Fruit needs to be eliminated in the healing phase of this diet. While there are healthy fruits, and I generally allow people to eat fruit even in my weight-loss plan, I am asking you to refrain from them in the first three-month healing phase of the cure.

The simple reason is that they contain sugar. Yes, it is all natural and does have some health benefits, but let's refrain from them for now. The sugar in the fruit, despite the fact that it is "all-natural," is the same bio-chemically as any of the other sugars I have mentioned. When your body is metabolizing the sugar, it doesn't matter where that sugar came from—ice cream or fruit.

Here is something else to consider about sugar. When you drink a 12-ounce glass of orange juice, you are consuming the juice of approximately six large oranges. That is an enormous amount of sugar—more than you would find in most sodas. Most of us would not consume that many oranges in one sitting, but we think nothing of drinking that much juice. Fruit juice is worse than fruit for you in the healing phase because there is so much more sugar in a glass of it than if you ate the actual fruit and you don't get any of the beneficial fiber.

I think that some fruits are better than others. For example, I encourage people to eat berries and melons rather than tropical fruits such as bananas and mangoes. I will discuss this in the transitional breathing-better phase of the program.

As an example, here is a quick list of the most common fruits and the amount of sugar found in each:

Apples (1 medium): 18 grams of sugar or 4.5 teaspoons

Bananas (1 medium): 18 grams of sugar or 4.5 teaspoons

Peaches (1 medium): 8 grams of sugar or 2 teaspoons

Plums (1 medium): 5 grams of sugar or 1 1/4 teaspoons

Nectarines (1 medium): 12 grams of sugar or 3 teaspoons

Oranges (1 medium): 16 grams of sugar or 4 teaspoons

Strawberries (1 cup): 9 grams of sugar or 2 1/4 teaspoons

Watermelon (1 cup): 12 grams of sugar or 3 teaspoons

However, no fruits are allowed in the healing phase of the diet program.

You can be surprised when you learn to really examine the food you are eating. Don't take anyone's word for it, especially someone who has a vested interest in having you consume certain products, such as the food manufacturing industry. Investigate food carefully before you eat it.

How to Use the Food Sensitivity Guides

The diet I am outlining in these diet chapters applies to everyone reading this book; therefore it is very general in which foods to eliminate. When you have your food sensitivity list, you must also eliminate those foods from your program. Since everyone's food sensitivity list will be different, I couldn't possibly give a specific diet for everyone. Eliminate a food to which you are sensitive, even if it is listed here as approved. Also, if there are foods that are negative in your food sensitivity chart and they are not listed here as allowed, you should not eat them. For example, if you tested negative for cane sugar, that doesn't mean you can eat it because I have just explained that you shouldn't. On the other hand, if I say in this chapter that it is acceptable to eat whole wheat yeast-free bread but you have a sensitivity to wheat, then you can't eat it.

Depending on the type of test you have had done, unless you did the general elimination technique, you should eliminate any of the foods in the two highest ranges of positiveness if you are an adult. If you are a child, or are doing this for your child, then anything that is not negative should be eliminated. If you did the general elimination technique, then anything that you suspect is a problem should be avoided from the permitted foods I list here.

It is easy to put the two of these together, and you must do that. That is the true basis for the diet part of the cure. One without the other will not work. Once you have completed the healing phase of the diet, your food sensitivities will begin to disappear. You do not have the same food sensitivities your whole life. And if you go through the healing phase, you may never have food sensitivities again. So just because I may be asking you to elimi-nate some of your favorite foods, it won't be forever—just until your body heals.

The Real Truth about Carbohydrates

There are so many myths about carbohydrates that I think this issue needs to be addressed. Just as all fats are not bad, the same is true for carbohydrates. There are simple carbohydrates and complex carbohydrates. Unless you wish to be on the weight-loss portion of this diet, you only need to eliminate the simple carbohydrates. The complex grains can be enjoyed by everyone, just on sliding scales, depending on whether you want to lose weight. I firmly believe in low-carbohydrate dieting, not no-carbohydrate dieting.

There have been many studies supporting the notion of healthy living through low-carbohydrate dieting. I think the message gets diluted and misrepresented when there are so many low-carbohydrate dieting books on the market that present one gimmick after another. One will tell you never to eat a carbohydrate again, but eat all the fat you want; another will tell you to eat only protein but then to eat all your carbohydrates during a certain time; and still another will tell you to find the right amount of carbohydrates for your body. None of them, except my book *Thin for Good,* teaches you how to eat them in just the right way so your body is metabolizing food the way it was designed to.

Please recall that we are genetically programmed to eat what grows in our environment and what we can catch and kill. That is just the way we have lived genetically for millions of years. It is only in the past century that we have begun to eat diets high in processed and refined foods. Only recently has the emphasis gone from fresh, whole foods to a diet that consists mainly of processed foods. There is an interesting study that looked at Third World peoples who were sheltered from Western eating habits. Once they were introduced to sugar, processed foods, and refined carbohydrates, their rates for heart disease and diabetes skyrocketed within one generation. We are now seeing the second wave of problems, which consists of allergies and asthma.

Low-carbohydrate diets have been linked to better cholesterol ratios, higher energy levels, lower risk for heart disease, lower risk for stroke, decreased mood swings, improved memory, and perhaps they may also help to keep you young. This is because low-carbohydrate diets help to regulate insulin, a very important hormone in the body. When you can control insulin levels, you can decrease your body's level of inflammation, help lower the number of anti-inflammatory medications you may need, and help yourself to breathe better.

There are three types of carbohydrates: sugar, starch, and fiber. Sugar and starch are the simple carbohydrates and are easily digested by the body. Fiber passes through the body relatively intact and helps to slow down the metabolism of food, allowing you to feel less hungry throughout the day and helping to regulate blood sugar and insulin levels.

Since we have already discussed one of the simple carbohydrates, sugar, let's now turn our attention to the starches. These also must be avoided. The foods in this category include most white foods: pasta, breads, pretzels, potatoes, rice cakes, white rice, parsnips, and most breakfast cereals, but especially puffed rice, puffed wheat, and corn flakes.

Highly refined grains cereals include:

- Basic 4
- Corn flakes
- Frosted flakes
- Just Right
- Kix
- Corn Pops
- Product 19
- Puffed Wheat
- Rice Krispies
- Special K
- Cream of Rice
- Cream of wheat or farina
- Grits
- Apple Jacks
- Instant oatmeal

Many other cereals can be included in this list. I have listed the most popular ones to give you an idea of things you should avoid. I suggest that you bring this book (me) along as a guide and incentive the first few times you start shopping under your new program.

Other foods in this category are peas, corn, tomatoes, and carrots. Although you may consider corn to be a vegetable, it is actually a starch. Peas are really legumes, and while most legumes are very healthy, peas are too starchy for the healing phase of this diet program. Carrots are not included simply because they are very high in sugar. Tomatoes are really a fruit and are to be avoided because of the sugar. I will discuss complex grains in the section where I discuss foods that are permissible for the cure.

The Evil Fungi: Candida and Yeast

There are a few simple things to help you remember what you should avoid:

- If it rises—it has yeast
- Anything with vinegar, such as mayonnaise and salad dressings
- Any edible fungi such as mushrooms, since they are molds themselves
- Any food that is fermented or contains a product of fermentation, such as soy sauce or tofu

You may also want to eliminate leftovers, since molds can grow pretty quickly on these foods, even if you don't see the mold itself. I am not suggesting that you throw leftovers away; simply freeze them immediately and heat them on another day. Other foods to be avoided include:

Dairy

Any kind of cheese, but especially the moldy, aged varieties such as Roquefort, must be avoided. The soft cheeses (cream, cottage, pot, farmer, and ricotta) generally do not contain much yeast, but do contain sugar, and that is why they should be avoided. In my prac-tice, if a patient is having a hard time with his or her diet, I do allow some of the soft cheeses, but in small amounts—up to 2 ounces per day. Sour cream, crème fraîche, and because of all the sugar in it, milk (fat-free, lactose-free, 1 percent, 2 percent—it is all the same in terms of sugar content) and yogurt (even unsweetened and sugar-free) should be avoided.

Condiments

These should be avoided because they contain vinegar. Examples include mayonnaise, mustard, soy sauce, monosodium glutamate (MSG—sometimes sold under the brand name Accent or Goya's Sazon), Worcestershire sauce, tamari, steak sauce, barbeque sauce, chili sauce, shrimp sauce, duck sauce, pickles, any pickled vegeta-bles, relishes, green olives, sauerkraut, horseradish, mincemeat, and store-bought salad dressings.

In my practice, I usually allow my patients to have mayonnaise and mustard. The amounts of vinegar in those two items, coupled with the amount you may be eating, are probably too low to cause much of a detriment to the program. This simple addition makes it a lot easier for most people to stay on their program; but, if you prefer to be a purist, then mayonnaise and mustard should be avoided as well. Also, salad dressings can be easily prepared at home by substi-tuting lemon juice or even lime juice for the vinegar.

Fermented Foods

Examples include smoked salmon (lox), smoked whitefish, tofu, and seitan. Be careful eating Japanese cuisine because much of the food is cured, and even the white rice in sushi contains sugar—it helps to make it sticky.

Malt Products

These include malted drinks such as Postum and Ovaltine, and most cereals. Malt is used in processing many processed foods and bever-ages. Beer is the best example in this category.

Alcohol

Alcohol is not permitted in the healing phase of the diet, to give your gut a chance to properly heal. They are also highly fermented beverages. Wine, vodka, gin, and almost all spirits contain sugar. However, the higher the alcohol content, the lower the amount of sugar.

Processed and Smoked Meats

Pickled or smoked meats and fish should be avoided due to the fermentation process. Bacon, ham, sausages, hot dogs, corned beef, salami, pastrami, and other similar meats also should be avoided. If you really like these foods and can't live without them, it is possible to find these meats uncured, and then they are allowed. The uncured versions are more expensive and do not last as long in your refrigerator, so be sure to freeze them if you think you may not be eating them so quickly. The processing and the smoking allow these meats to last a long time. If they remain uncured, these meats can go bad very quickly, and you may not know that if you are a first-time buyer.

Edible Fungi

These include mushrooms of any variety, morels, and truffles.

There are many foods that contain yeast, but do not get discouraged because soon we will be discussing all the foods you can be eating. Here is a list I give my patients just so you get a quick idea of what to avoid. Make a copy of this, shrink it, and keep it in your purse or wallet so you can always refer to it.

Foods to be avoided on a yeast-free diet include:

- Alcoholic beverages
- All foods that contain sugar
- Barbecue sauce
- Biscuits
- Breads
- Buttermilk
- Candy
- Catsup
- Cereals
- Cheese
- Cookies
- Cottage cheese
- Crackers
- Dried and cured foods
- Dried fruits
- Dry roasted nuts
- Fermented beverages
- Flour
- Frozen or canned fruit or juices

- Hamburger and hot dog buns
- Horseradish
- Mayonnaise
- Milk
- Mushrooms
- Olives (green)
- Pastries
- Pickles
- Root beer
- Rolls
- Sauerkraut
- Smoked foods
- Soy sauce
- Store-bought dressings
- Teas
- Tomato sauce
- Truffles
- Vinegar

Avoid the following yeast-containing flour products and foods (read the labels carefully):

- Yeasted breads
- Crackers
- Biscuits
- Pretzels
- Rolls
- Hamburger and hot dog buns
- Pastries
- Pancakes
- Breaded fish or chicken
- Mushrooms

Avoid fermented foods and products that contain fermented foods:

- Cheese
- Vinegar
- Salad dressings
- Alcoholic beverages and nonalcoholic wine and beer
- Mayonnaise
- Soy sauce
- Tamari
- Sour cream
- Crème fraîche
- Sauerkraut
- Fermented beverages
- Olives

- Pickles
- Dry roasted nuts

Avoid all sugars and foods containing sugars:

- White sugar, brown sugar, corn syrup, fruit juices, etc.
- Cookies, candy, cake, ice cream, soda, pies, puddings
- Fruits
- Dried fruits
- Catsup
- Malted products
- Milk

These are handy reference guides; see the full explanations of these categories to ensure that you are following the diet program correctly. I know this seems like a lot of work. Almost all of my patients feel the same way when I first explain things to them, but after a week or so, they no longer feel deprived and are feeling so much better that it is all worth it.

Now it's time to explain all the delicious foods you can eat.

Foods to Eat in the Healing Phase

Whether you wish to lose weight or not, you need to read this section. The rules I am about to outline apply for every person wishing to take part in the cure. This is not as strict as you might think, nor is it as rigorous as the weight-loss part of the program. In this section I want everyone to become comfortable with the permitted foods. Once that takes place, you can learn how to modify this program so you can lose weight, too, if that's what you want or need to do. Just to reassure the thin people reading this book, you are probably going to lose a few pounds. That is inevitable because sugar makes us retain water. So even the thinnest person can expect to lose up to 5 pounds simply by eliminating sugar. However, once your body adjusts to the new way of eating, you can put those pounds back on by eating correctly.

This healing phase will probably last about three months. It may last up to six months if you do not follow the guidelines as you should. If perfect, by the end of the third month, you will be able to start increasing the choices in your diet and reintroducing new foods. I will teach you how to do that in the breathing-better phase of the cure.

In a program designed for allergy and asthma treatment, the issue of inflammation needs to be addressed. I have mentioned this repeatedly. Our diets are one of the main sources of inflammation that we face daily. By following this program, you will be ridding your body of a main source of inflammation. For example, if cats triggered an asthma attack for you (and you weren't already a cat owner), would you have cats in your house? The same holds for foods. We eat at least three times per day, and that repetitive level of inflammation needs to be addressed if you are ever to get off some of your medications and breathe more easily.

The healing phase is meant to help your body get rid of all the inflammation that has been accumulating for years. I know three months seems like a long time, but that is the only way to truly start to heal. Chronic inflammation takes a long time to improve. Six to eight weeks is considered the minimum time to heal any acute muscular injury. The level of inflammation that any person with asthma or allergies has endured has lasted for a significant period, and it is going to take a significant amount of time to bring the level of inflammation in your body back down to normal. That is not to say that it is going to take that long for you to start to feel better. Quite the contrary—it may only take a week or two for you to start noticing improvements. I am confident that your need for medication will start to lessen in this short period of time, but don't reduce anything without discussing it first with your doctor.

This diet program is designed to decrease inflammation in several ways. The first is by increasing the amounts of omega-3 fatty acids and decreasing the amount of omega-6 fatty acids that you consume. Also, this cure will begin to change what your body has been using for fuel for many years. You will stop using simple carbohydrates for energy and instead use what we were intended to use for fuel—complex carbohydrates, proteins, and healthy fats. These are much more efficient sources of fuel, and your metabolism is going to start working better and faster because that is what it is meant to work on. The second way is by eliminating all of the foods that have yeast or that feed the yeast that you already have, living overgrown throughout your body. To do this will be a fun challenge, but if you are like my patients, you will be happy and relieved to finally be doing something to control your breathing and to feel better.

What Can I Eat?

Following are the allowable foods for anyone taking this cure. I am not going to discuss portion control until we get to the weight-loss portion of the program. I believe that portions are not that relevant if you are eating the correct foods. The beauty of this program is that there is nothing to count—carbohydrate grams, fat grams, or calories. By eating the proper foods, your body's metabolism will be operating at its peak level of efficiency and you won't have to concern yourself with counting anything. Just focus on getting the allowable foods correct and ensuring that your diet remains varied. A varied diet is important because I do not want you to develop new food sensitivities while we are trying to cure the ones you already have. I am going to list the foods by category to serve as a quick reference guide.

Eat as much as you want of anything listed as long as each meal contains 55 percent proteins and 45 percent complex carbohydrates. If you want to lose weight, read this chapter first and get to know the foods you can pick from. The weight-loss program will differ by focusing on the quantity of each category of food vis-à-vis the protein-to-carbohydrate ratio. So whether you need or want to lose weight or not, this is the right place to start.

Getting the correct ratio is relatively simple. Just look at your plate at each meal. If there is more protein on it than anything else, then you have reached this ratio. This must be done at each meal. For example, don't eat a heavy, carbohydrate-laden breakfast and make up for it by only eating protein the rest of the day. That won't work metabolically. Each meal must have the proper ratio. But don't get caught up measuring this; use a rough estimate. If you start trying to be exact, you are going to get bogged down in the unimportant aspects of the cure. Most important is to have more protein on your plate than complex carbohydrates at each meal; then you will have satisfied this requirement. Focus on the types of food, not the amount.

Just learn what you may eat, and if you need or want to lose weight, we will worry about quantities in chapter 9.

Proteins

These are going to be your main source of food for the next three to six months. They are great sources of fuel, and the yeast cannot feed on them. Protein is important for many of the body's functions, including tissue growth, immune system regulation (vital in this case), muscular strength and tone, proper digestion, and the formation of hormones. Proteins activate glucagon, the hormone that assists us in losing weight, building lean muscle mass, stabilizing energy levels, controlling hunger, and decreasing inflammation caused by an over-abundance of insulin. Therefore, your appetite will be normalized and your food cravings will disappear, so don't be afraid to eat this very important category of food. However, due to certain health considerations, I would like to help you learn how to eat these not only in a yeast-free way, but in a health-conscious way as well.

Red Meats

All red meats are permissible in the healing phase of the diet. These include beef, veal, lamb, pork, rabbit, venison, and other game animals. Game animals tend to have less fat than farm-raised animals. To maintain the integrity of the diet, that is all you need to know. However, there are some extra hints you should be aware of if you want to follow this program in as healthy a way as possible.

1. Cook the meat with the fat intact, if you prefer, but I recommend trimming the fat before eating. Animals, just as we do, store all their toxins and any antibiotic residue in their fat cells. Why eat this? On a yeast-free diet, we want to avoid antibiotics in any way we can, and when we eat commercial meats, we are getting the antibiotic residues the animals ingest, especially if we consume the fat. Fat in the muscle of the meat itself is fine; it is the excess fat that I am asking you to avoid. A recent study blames the antibiotics that our livestock eat for the fact that bacteria we come into contact with are becoming resistant to antibiotics.

2. In the same vein, I recommend that you try to eat as organically as possible. While that may not be possible or cost-effective for you, keep in mind that organically raised animals should be free of any antibiotics, growth hormones, or diseases.

3. Processed meats are a big issue for some people because they are used by low-carbohydrate advocates encouraging their clients to eat all the bacon they want. However, bacon is mostly the wrong kind of fat—saturated fat. Most other processed meats have nitrates, nitrites, and sugar in them as part of the curing process. They also contain chemical preservatives that we should avoid. I am not advocating that you avoid these altogether, just eat them with restraint, and steer more toward the meats such as turkey or roast beef, since usually they are not processed.

Fish

There are no limitations to the kind or amount of fish or other seafood. Permitted fish include but are not limited to tuna, salmon, swordfish, herring, pompano, mahi-mahi, catfish, trout, sole, cod, flounder, bluefish, sea bass, and tilapia. Shellfish include but are not limited to shrimp, scallops, lobster, conch, calamari, clams, oysters, mussels, abalone, squid, and crab.

I encourage my patients to eat a lot of their protein from this category. Fish are high in omega-3 fatty acids, which are known to decrease inflammation. Fish also contain one of the heart-healthiest oils you can consume. However, there are certain ways to ensure that this category of food is as healthy as it can be:

1. Be careful that the fish you eat are not farm-raised unless you know that the farm raises healthy fish. Fish that are farm-raised may be kept in unhealthy and unsanitary conditions. Most fish are organically grown—they are caught in the wild. Farm fish may not be as pure, since they are fed things they would normally not eat if they were wild, and they are usually given antibiotics. Be careful to choose only fish that have been caught in the wild.

2. Try to limit the larger fish you eat. Again, this is simply for health reasons. The larger the fish, the more mercury it may contain, because they eat more small fish. Shellfish, since they tend to live on the bottom of the ocean, may also contain high levels of mer-

cury since mercury is a heavy metal and falls to the bottom of the ocean. Fish are the second-largest source of mercury toxicity in the world; dental fillings are the principal cause.

Poultry

All poultry is permissible. This includes but is not limited to chickens, turkeys, ducks, Cornish hens, pheasants, quails, and guinea hens. Some caveats for health include:

1. Try to eat organically raised chicken. Nonorganic fowl contains growth hormones and antibiotics.
2. Commercially raised chickens are force-fed and live in harsh conditions that stimulate the release in their bodies of stress hormones that are probably best left uneaten. This may even give the meat a bad taste. The bird is the sum of what it eats and how it is killed.
3. Avoid eating poultry skin, since it is where the animal deposits its antibiotic residue and any toxins.
4. Try to eat more white meat than dark, since white meat has less fat.

Eggs

These are a great source of protein and also make wonderful snacks that can be eaten on the run. Although eggs have gotten a bad reputation, many studies have shown no correlation between the amount of eggs you consume and your cholesterol level. By themselves, eggs do not raise your cholesterol. Almost all of the egg's nutritional value is in the yolk. When cooking eggs to enjoy, unless the recipe calls for it (such as in a meringue), never eat the egg white without the yolk. The yolk of the egg contains lecithin, which is a natural cholesterol-lowering agent. And never eat egg substitutes. In a landmark study, rats that were fed only egg substitutes died of malnutrition. There is simply no health benefit from egg substitutes. To make your egg eating even healthier, follow these tips:

1. If you purchase nothing else that is organic, please purchase and eat organic eggs when you can. There is a huge difference in the chemical composition between organic and nonorganic eggs. Organic eggs are not that much more expensive and usually are

found in most supermarkets. Organic eggs contain omega-3 and omega-6 fatty acids in the ratio that nature intended them to have: 1 to 1. Commercially raised eggs contain nineteen times more omega-6 fatty acids than omega-3s. This is what I believe makes commercially raised eggs unhealthy—not the cholesterol in them. Besides, one of the main premises of the cure is to reduce the amount of omega-6 fatty acids in our diet. This is one way. To my knowledge, there has never been a study to prove that by eating cholesterol, your cholesterol will go up.

2. Ensure that the egg yolk you do consume is thoroughly cooked. This will decrease your risk for contracting salmonella, which is rampant in commercially raised chickens and their eggs. If you buy organic eggs, your risk for contracting salmonella is decreased. Salmonella is the primary reason why commercially raised hens are given antibiotics and organic ones are not.

Cheese

This is an easy category because these are not permitted in the healing phase of the diet program.

Fats

Since so many people are still convinced that all fats are bad for them, this is probably a good place to lay most of those fears to rest. While a higher-protein diet is certainly higher in fat than the American Heart Association calls for, not only doesn't it have to be if you choose the correct proteins, but also there are no definitive studies to say that a low-fat diet is healthy. There has been only one study done to prove that a low-fat diet is healthy. The Ornish diet is the only diet that has been proven to reverse heart disease. In that diet, less than 10 percent of your daily food consumption is fat. That program also emphasizes such things as meditation. While it may reverse heart disease in some instances, it is an extremely difficult diet for most people to follow over an extended period of time. It is my firm belief that the popularization of this type of diet has led to the obesity epidemic in the United States.

Another recent study showed that diets with more than 30 percent of their calories from fat were healthier than those with 10 to 30 percent of their calories from fat—the American Heart Association (AHA) recommendation. Yet there is blind faith that a low-fat diet is the healthiest. It is just not true and has never been proven. By the same token, there have never been any studies to show that a low-carbohydrate diet posed any significant health risks. In fact, a Mediterranean-type diet similar to the one I am asking you to follow has been shown time and again to be healthy, yet it is not espoused by the AHA.

The Types of Fat.   There are essentially three types of fat: saturated, monounsaturated, and polyunsaturated.

Saturated Fats.   At room temperature, these fats are solid or semisolid. These are the types of fat found in red meats and tropical oils. Most consumers think these are unhealthy, yet the tropical oils are both antibacterial and antifungal. Two-thirds of the saturated fats in these oils are the short- and medium-chain fatty acids, which are healthy. In fact, lauric acid is an example of these types of fat found in coconut oil and in human breast milk—if it is good for an infant, it is probably good for us as adults.

Conjugated linoleic acid (CLA) is a medium-chain fatty acid in red meat. It cannot be obtained from any other dietary source, and preliminary studies show this to be cancer-protective, aid in the prevention of heart disease, boost the immune system, and decrease body fat.

Monounsaturated Fats.   These are some of the healthiest oils you can use. Good examples of these are olive oil and macadamia nut oil. Olive oil and macadamia nut oil are the best oils to use for anything, and macadamia nut oil is my personal favorite. Olive oil contains 73 percent monounsaturated fat and is almost completely neutral—meaning it contains mostly omega-9 fatty acids. Macadamia nut oil is 80 to 85 percent monounsaturated fat, making it the most heart-healthy, with the least amount of omega-6 fatty acids. The omega-6 fatty acid content is 8 percent for olive oil, only 3 percent for macadamia nut oil, and 25 percent for canola oil. Both olive oil and macadamia nut oil have high smoke points, but olive oil's is 200°F and macadamia nut oil's is 410°F—making macadamia nut oil a much safer and healthier choice. It has taken over from olive oil as my new favorite because of these characteristics. I suggest that everyone try this oil and use it liberally; it gives food a light, nutty flavor.

I wish I could recommend canola oil, which, if used at all, should only be used *cold*. Never heat canola oil because it turns rancid when heated. That means it becomes all transfatty acids, which are extremely unhealthy. When heated, canola oil has a worse chemical makeup than margarine. Use macadamia nut oil for cooking and salad dressings, olive oil for Italian food recipes, and relegate canola oil to the trash.

Polyunsaturated Fats.   These are the fats most of us consume daily. They include corn, safflower, soybean, cottonseed, sunflower, peanut, fish, and flaxseed oils. These are the omega-6 fatty acids I have been discussing. Omega-3 and omega-6 fats are considered essential because they cannot be produced by our bodies and must be ingested. Therefore, not all omega-6 fats are bad. It is just that our diets are extremely high in omega-6 fatty acids and not high enough in omega-3s. If you eat any processed foods, you are getting enough of the omega-6 fats.

Omega-3 and omega-6 fatty acids should be balanced in the preferred healthy 1 to 1 ratio. That usually does not happen, because omega-6 fats are in most processed foods and most foods prepared out-side the home, including fast foods. Many researchers believe that those with diets high in omega-6 fatty acids suffer from higher levels of inflammation, which may eventually lead to allergies, asthma, arthritis, psoriasis, eczema, and irritable bowel, to name several ailments.

Omega-3 fatty acids have been proposed to promote better health by decreasing inflammation. They are believed to positively affect blood pressure, enhance the immune system, and decrease the inci-dence of heart disease. This is why it is critical to eat a diet that has the proper balance of these two main components. All fats are not bad, and we need to make better choices in the fats we eat, rather than trying to eliminate fats from our diet altogether.

Transfatty Acids.   This is the last category of fats to discuss and perhaps the deadliest. These are formed during hydrogenation, a process that allows these oils, foods, and fats to have a longer shelf life—good for the manufacturer, but not so good for us. They are com-posed of an altered chemical molecule that occurs during the heating or manipulation of a food that contains fat. This usually occurs during the processing. Transfatty acids are commonly found in margarine, solid vegetable shortening, commercially baked goods such as cookies and chips, and most prepared foods. Anything that reads "partially hydrogenated" on a food label is a transfatty acid. The type of oil is irrelevant—it is the hydrogenation that we need to stay away from.

Transfats are believed to be the primary cancer-causing agent in fats. I never recommend using margarine or solid vegetable shortening for this reason. Margarine contains up to 25 percent transfatty acids and heated canola oil contains up to 75 percent transfats, depending on how much you heat it.

When it comes to fats and oils, the simpler you can make it, the better. Use macadamia nut oil exclusively if you can, especially when heating it. Use olive oil for Italian food recipes if you have run out of macadamia nut oil, and never use canola oil. Avoid margarine and any other oil that is partially hydrogenated.

To make your program even healthier, use these tips when thinking about oils:

1. Always try to buy oils that have been cold and expeller pressed. These oils tend to undergo less hydrogenation because they are made into oils under less harsh conditions.
2. Try to avoid oils that have any preservatives in them, such as BHT. If the oil is good, it should not need any preservatives.
3. Last, store your oil in a cool, dark place, and buy oils in dark containers. This helps the oil maintain its integrity and not convert into anything unhealthy.

Dr. Frank Sacks, a cardiac researcher from the Harvard School of Public Health, said, "We've made some mistakes with the low-fat message." He explained that it led many people to adopt a poor dietary pattern and to consume a diet loaded with refined carbohydrates. The results have been poor nutrition, widespread weight gain, a large rise in diabetes, and little or no benefit to the heart. Please keep these in mind when you are concerned about consuming protein. We need a new approach, and since diet involves so many factors, it is hard to isolate one thing that will make the difference. I believe that if we stick to whole, unprocessed foods, we are bound to be healthier.

Complex Carbohydrates

The biggest thing to keep in mind about this category is that it includes fruits, complex grains, and vegetables. Most Americans associate breads and pasta with carbohydrates, but there are many delicious carbohydrates we tend to overlook. Complex carbohydrates are the only carbohydrates allowed in the healing phase of this program. As I mentioned before, fruits, because of their sugar content, are not allowed for the first three months. Here is what is allowed:

Vegetables

This group is divided into several subgroups, depending on the carbohydrate amount in the vegetable. This is not that important for the person who does not need or who does not want to lose weight, but is for the person who wishes to drop some weight.

The lowest-carbohydrate group includes salad vegetables, which are less than 10 percent carbohydrates. These include green, leafy vegetables such as iceberg, romaine, Boston, and Bibb lettuces; escarole; kale; beet greens; Swiss chard; collard greens; dandelion; parsley; spinach; mustard greens; endive; arugula; and bok choy. Fennel, celery, radishes, peppers, bean sprouts, and cucumbers also are in this group. There are many other forms of lettuce or leafy vegetable that would be included here as well. You may eat these raw, cooked, frozen, or fresh. Although iceberg lettuce is the most consumed vegetable in this country, it probably has the least amount of nutritive value—it is mostly water. Try to eat the darker sections of the lettuce or the darker greens such as spinach if you can. The amount of these vegetables that you can consume is unlimited.

The second subgroup constitutes the vegetables that are between 10 and 25 percent carbohydrates. This is a much longer list and includes most of the vegetables. These include broccoli, cauliflower, turnips, eggplant, asparagus, avocados, snow pea pods, cabbage, Brussels sprouts, scallions, leeks, onions, water chestnuts, summer squash (zucchini), spaghetti squash, okra, artichoke hearts, string beans, garlic, shallots, and most other vegetables. Generally, if the vegetable is not named in the first or the third subgroup, then it is in this group. The amount of these vegetables you can consume is unlimited.

The third subgroup of vegetables is the highest in carbohydrate content. The ones that are available to be eaten in the healing phase of the program include parsnips, winter squash (butternut, buttercup, or acorn), sweet potatoes, celery roots, and artichokes. Nonpermissible foods in this group include white potatoes, beets, peas, carrots, tomatoes, and corn. Ethnic root vegetables also are in this category and include jicama, breadfruit, christophene, cassava, and plantains. These vegetables should be limited to 1 cup, cooked, three times per week.

Grains

The only grains allowed in the healing phase of the diet are the complex ones. All simple carbohydrates are metabolized in the body the same way as sugar. Therefore these need to be avoided, as I explained earlier.

When choosing a grain product, always look at the ingredients list. Look for the word "whole" before any grain. This can be wheat, oat, rye, seven-grain, etc. It must have "whole" in front or it is not whole grain bread—even if the label says it is whole grain. (That is another food manufacturing trick that does nothing but confuse the public.) The same holds true for cereals. Even the healthiest-looking cereals with the nicest packaging can be nothing more than well-disguised simple carbohydrates. Ensure that there is no yeast in the ingredients list, too. You must read the ingredients lists or you will never know for sure.

The grains in this category are brown rice (white rice and risotto are simple grains), barley, oats, wheat, buckwheat (kasha), spelt, soy flour, kamut, teff, milo, amaranth, corn, and quinoa. Although some of these grains may sound foreign to you, they are becoming more and more readily available, even in regular supermarket chains.

If you are going to eat bread in this category, it must say "yeast-free" on the label; check the ingredients list if you aren't sure. Most crackers are made from simple grains, and I have yet to find a cracker that I think is acceptable in this phase of the diet. Ry-vita is an example of an acceptable crackerlike product that does not contain yeast and is a whole grain. A common mistake some of my patients make is to eat pita or matzoh. While those products are yeast-free grains, they are usually simple carbohydrates and should be avoided in the healing phase.

Pastas.   Most familiar pastas and certainly those you would eat out are refined and simple carbohydrates and are not permitted in the healing phase of the diet. This includes the Jerusalem artichoke and vegetable pasta varieties. However, whole-grain pastas are available made from brown rice (usually too sticky if overcooked), whole wheat, spelt, quinoa, kamut, soy, and even corn. These are all best and taste more like regular pasta when undercooked. Again, please refer to the ingredients list to ensure that the pasta you choose is made from a whole grain. Another helpful hint (this would apply to any grain product): If the label or ingredients list says it is an enriched product, then it is a simple carbohydrate. There would be no need to enrich the food if it were a complex, whole grain. Pasta does not contain yeast.

This category of food is permissible up to 1 cup, cooked, three times per week in the healing phase of the diet. Certain additional restrictions apply to the person who desires to lose weight, and those are found in chapter 9.

Grains That May Be Eaten on a Yeast-Free Diet

Whole grains: Brown rice (short-, medium-, or long-grain, not wild), cracked wheat, Bulgar wheat, millet, oats, barley, buckwheat (kasha), quinoa, amaranth, teff, and spelt.

Breads: Anything that is yeast-free and is whole-grain, such as sourdough, rye, essene, spelt, kamut, and ezekiel.

Cereals: Hot wheat, oatmeal (not instant), brown rice, mixed whole grain, puffed millet, corn, rice, wheat, quinoa, and kashi.

Pasta: Whole wheat, udon, corn, brown rice, and buckwheat (Soba).

As you can see, there are many healthy, complex carbohydrates you may eat while in the healing phase of the diet. I limit the highest-carbohydrate foods so that your body truly starts to heal from the many years of inflammation. The limits will also help you to keep to the 55–45 rule.

Legumes

This is a very healthy part of the food chain that many of us forget about. This category includes lentils, kidney beans, black beans, lima beans, fava beans, black-eyed peas, navy beans, and peanuts. These are excellent sources of fiber and many nutrients and are great nonanimal sources of protein. Bean products such as tofu and tempeh are also in this category but are not permissible because they are fermented. This category of foods is allowed up to 1 cup, cooked, three times per week.

An important side note is that whenever I am limiting the categories of food, I encourage my patients not to eat them on the same day. For example, have whole grains on one day, legumes on another, and the higher-carbohydrate vegetables on another day. This keeps your diet varied and the all-important 55–45 rule easy to follow. Also, I set upper limits as to the amount of food you are allowed. You do not have to eat all the permissible foods on any given day.

Nuts and Seeds

These are very important and should be part of every healthy diet. Although they are high in fat, they contain good, heart-healthy oils. The nuts and seeds you may eat include pecans, walnuts, almonds, Brazil nuts, cashews, filberts, pumpkin seeds, sunflower seeds, macadamia nuts, and pistachios. The only nut not included in this category is peanuts. They are legumes and are listed in that section.

Nut butters are included in this category, too. These include almond, cashew, macadamia nut butters, and all nut butters except peanut butter. They are delicious and usually all-natural, and I recommend them highly. The permissible amount is 3 tablespoons per day.

To include even healthier foods in this category, I recommend that you buy fresh, unroasted nuts. This tends to make them less susceptible to contamination with any mold. It is also believed that peanuts and pistachios have the most mold contamination and should be avoided. However, I allow my patients to eat any kind of nut they want, within the permissible guidelines, and have found that restricting these two items is clinically unnecessary, and is only for the purist.

The recommended amount of nuts or seeds to eat in one day is 2 ounces. This is not an enormous amount of nuts or seeds—about 20. I suggest that you buy nuts in 1-ounce packages, or if that becomes too costly, then buy them in larger quantities and then parcel them out yourself before you get hungry, to make sure you can stay within the guidelines.

Extras

What is a diet without a bonus that you didn't expect? The two things that many of my patients like to use as snacks are olives and avocados.

Both of these foods are very high in good, heart-healthy fats. This serves two purposes. The first is that they are nutritionally dense foods that make great snacks and additions to other meals, such as salads. Second, because of their high fat content, they keep you satiated and less hungry throughout the day. Please limit yourself to 4 olives per day and 1 avocado.

Protein Bars/Shakes

This is a booming part of the health food market right now. In the past few years, with the surging popularity of low-carbohydrate diets, many new products have been advertised as low-carb. These include shakes, bars, candy, muffins, and bagels, among many others. I noticed that those who ate these tended to have more difficulty staying on their diet. I always assumed it was because these things simulated foods that should not be part of a dieter's repertoire. For example, if you are trying to lose weight, or have a weight problem, you should probably learn how to live without candy-type snacks. I would recommend these products as meal replacements, not as snacks—the way many people use them.

The real truth has recently been uncovered. ConsumerLab recently released a report saying that many of the health bar labels misstate the level of carbohydrates they contain. Eighteen companies, including many well-known ones, were involved in this devious marketing procedure. They did not count the glycerin, polydextrose, xylitol, or other sweeteners in their count.

The labels have all been corrected for accuracy. However, I would use this caution: Be very wary of low-carbohydrate grain products. When I was the Associate Medical Director of the Atkins Center in NYC, we independently tested one low-carbohydrate bagel that claimed to have 3 grams of carbohydrate and found it to have 55 grams instead. I therefore recommend that most people refrain from products of this sort.

With proper high-protein, low-carbohydrate products available, I suggest you limit these to the following portions:

Protein bars: Try to use these only as meal replacements. Limit your use to 1 to 2 per day maximum. Use these as snacks only if desperately hungry.

Or

Protein shakes: These are quite convenient to use, especially for breakfast or as a snack after work or school. Most of them taste quite good and need only to be mixed with water. One patient recently taught me a trick—add a tablespoon of peanut butter to the shake mixture, place it in a blender, and the shake becomes much thicker. I suggest no more than 2 shakes per day and always try to use these as a meal replacement, rather than a snack. People who are sensitive or allergic to milk should avoid these, since most of them are made from whey protein, which is made from milk.

Or

High-protein candy bars: There are many currently available on the market. I suggest you limit your use to 2 servings per day. The serving size is usually quite small, so please be careful to check into that before indulging in an entire bar.

With the products in this category, choose ones that are less than 4 to 6 grams of carbohydrate per serving. Please pay attention to the serving size; most are quite small to keep the carbohydrate counts low. You may mix and match these products as long as you stay within the recommended maximum amount. I do *not* suggest you have 2 servings of each of these per day. They are an optional indulgence; eat these sparingly, if at all. Always try to eat real, whole foods when possible.

Condiments/Butter/Oils

Please check the ingredients list of any condiment that you wish to use, especially if it is bottled or if it is a combination spice product. Some may contain sugar, which must be avoided in this program. The two biggest condiment offenders are margarine and ketchup, which must be avoided entirely in the healing phase of the program.

Spices: Most spices, unless they contain monosodium glutamate or any other preservative, are permissible in unlimited amounts in the healing phase.

Butter/ghee: This is permissible up to 3 tablespoons per day.

Macadamia nut oil: This is the preferred oil and is permissible in unlimited quantities. Olive oil is allowed, too, in unlimited quantities.

Mayonnaise/mustard: Although purists would tell you to avoid these because of the vinegar, if you keep to 3 tablespoons of each per day, you should not have any problems, and your vinegar intake will be minimal.

Vinegar: This must be avoided except as noted above.

Lemon/lime juice: This is permissible up to 6 teaspoons per day. It is great to mix with oil to make salad dressings, since vinegar is not permitted except as noted above.

Beverages

Water. This is the gold standard for drinking. I encourage you to use this as your sole beverage. As we age, we become chronically dehydrated. We get so used to not drinking water that our bodies learn to turn off our thirst mechanism. We get so consumed with drinking other beverages that we forget to drink the most important: water. Even if you don't feel thirsty, it is still important to drink water.

Water is essential to life. It helps regulate body temperature, cushion joints, remove toxins (very important for this process), maintain strength and endurance, protect organs and tissues, and carry nutrients to every cell in the body. By the time you are actually thirsty, you are already mildly dehydrated. Some common symptoms of chronic dehydration are headache, fatigue, flushed skin, light-headedness, and dry mouth.

It is believed that during chronic dehydration, the body produces more histamine—exactly what we are trying to avoid. Histamine can regulate the thirst mechanism. The spasms that histamine incites in the bronchial tubes are actually an attempt to conserve water. Dehydration also may account for the runny noses and watery eyes that accompany allergies. To cope with pollens and other antigens, histamines and other chemicals, direct water to the eyes and nose to remove the offending allergens. Therefore, it is critical to drink the necessary amounts of water per day.

My rule of thumb is that you should drink a little less than half your body weight in ounces of water per day. My official rule is to divide your weight by 2.2 pounds to get your weight in kilograms—that is the amount of water in ounces that you should be drinking. For example, if you weigh 220 pounds, divide that by 2.2 and you weigh 100 kilograms; therefore, you should drink 100 ounces of water per day. This total does not include any other beverage except herbal tea or club soda. Everything else that you drink does not count in the total. The water may be tap, filtered, spring, bottled, or carbonated. However, if you exercise, you should add 16 ounces to the total for every 45 minutes of a strenuous activity such as running. For every ounce of caffeinated beverage that you drink, you need to drink an additional 2 ounces of water.

Soda.   Diet soda is permitted in the healing phase of the diet. This holds true for all other low-calorie beverages, carbonated or not. I feel that soda should be avoided in the interest of health. Most soda products are highly noxious beverages. They are filled with chemicals (diet sodas are filled with even more) and have no nutritional value. However, if you must have soda, try to limit its use to no more than 24 ounces per day of a diet beverage.

Coffee/Tea.   The beverage I recommend in this category is herbal tea, and the amount is unlimited. However, consumption of coffee or tea, whether or not it is decaffeinated, will not hinder your process of healing, provided you replace the water. I recommend that you consume coffee and tea in moderation; the true yeast-free diet advocates would eliminate consumption of these two beverages completely, because mold can enter in the processing of the tea leaves or coffee beans. With all the other consumption restrictions in the program, this may prove to be too hard for some people. I therefore ask my patients to limit these to 2 cups per day, maximum. In the interests of best health, eliminate coffee and tea completely.

Milk. This is forbidden in the healing phase of the diet. Skim, whole, 2 percent, 1 percent, and lactose-free milk are all the same in one respect—they contain equal amounts of sugar. Heavy cream may be used in moderation, up to 3 tablespoons per day. This can be watered down to use in your yeast-free cereal and it will be just like milk, only healthier. Heavy cream also can be used in recipes as a thickening agent or in your coffee. Don't make mistakes in this category. Heavy cream is preferable, but light cream may be used, too, but not half and half (it is half milk).

Unsweetened soy or rice milk may be used up to 4 ounces per day. Again, it is important that you read the labels of these two products closely. Most of them contain more sugar than regular milk. Be especially wary of the vanilla or other flavored varieties. It must have fewer than 4 grams of sugar per serving to be acceptable for the healing phase of this program.

Alcohol. This category is prohibited in this phase of the diet. But, if you must indulge, please avoid wine and beer at all costs. Vodka and scotch are the two most acceptable forms of liquor in this program. If you are attending a special occasion, then please make sure that it is one of these two—have them straight or mixed with club soda. Avoid tonic, unless it is diet, as it has more sugar than soda. Also, never mix these with fruit juices.

Fruits

These are not permitted in the healing phase of the diet. The same applies to fruit juices.

Desserts

The quick answer is that these must be avoided. However, diet gelatin is a commercially available dessert that will not upset the healing phase of the diet. There are probably other desserts that you can make with stevia, saccharin, or Splenda that can work. Please refer to *Thin For Good*, or any of the many low-carbohydrate cookbooks for recommendations.

As you can see, there are many foods available to eat. I have been very successful with patients following this diet. They were able to reduce or rid themselves of medications and were able to breathe better. I know it could help you, too.

Whenever I am creating a diet for patients or for readers of my other books, I like to teach them what foods to eat so they may then create what they like to eat. Eating is an individual pursuit, and our tastes vary. I hope this chapter gives you the necessary tools to create a delicious world of eating for the next three months. You will feel better in the process.

The rules in this chapter apply to everyone who wants to be part of the cure—whether they have weight issues or not. In the next chapter I will teach you how to adapt this program if you want to lose weight along the way.

The Allergy and Asthma Cure Step Four: Review

1. Make a true commitment to the program.
2. Decide which healing-phase diet you are going to follow—weight loss or regular.
3. Have a list of your food sensitivities handy.
4. Clean out your cabinets and refrigerator of anything not permissible on this program.
5. Fill out a symptom questionnaire; place it aside for two weeks, then reassess every two weeks for a total of three months.
6. Begin the cure.
7. Eliminate sugar from your diet.
8. Eliminate any fruit or fruit juice.
9. Eliminate any food on your food sensitivity list from the two highest levels of positiveness if you are an adult.
10. If you are doing this program for a child, then any food that tested positive, no matter how positive, should be eliminated.
11. If you did the general elimination diet technique, then any suspect food should be eliminated.

12. Even though the food appears on the permissible list in this chapter, if it appears positive in your food sensitivity chart, it must be avoided.
13. If the food is negative on the food sensitivity list but not on the permissible list, you cannot have it.
14. Eliminate simple carbohydrates and starches. Refer to the list if you have to—that is what it is here for. Simple rule: If it is white and processed, it is best avoided.
15. Eliminate any fermented foods.
16. Avoid vinegar.
17. Avoid cheese.
18. Avoid smoked meats or fish.
19. Avoid mushrooms.
20. If not on a weight-loss plan, then simply make each meal have 55 percent proteins and 45 percent complex carbohydrates. Simply, slightly more protein than anything else.
21. Don't focus on the amount of food, but on the types of food.
22. Use organic eggs if you buy nothing else organic.
23. Use macadamia nut oil exclusively if you can. Olive oil is the next best choice.
24. Use other oils sparingly and never use margarine or canola oil.
25. Refer to the vegetable list—unlimited use of the first two sub-groups and 1 cup, cooked, three times per week of the third subgroup.
26. Eat only complex grains—1 cup, cooked, three times per week.
27. If you are going to eat bread, then it must say "yeast-free" on the label.
28. Legumes are allowed up to 1 cup, cooked, three times per week.
29. Of the food categories that are limited, try not to eat them on the same day.
30. Rotate and vary your food choices.
31. Nuts or seeds are allowable up to 2 ounces per day.
32. Drink your body weight in pounds divided by 2 in ounces of water each day.
33. Limit high-protein shakes/bars/candy to 2 servings per day of either; try to use them as meal replacements, not snacks.
34. Avoid high-protein grain products.
35. Try to avoid caffeine.

36. Alcohol is not permitted except on special occasions; vodka and scotch, either straight or with club soda, are the preferred choices.
37. Don't forget to keep your symptom questionnaire.

9

The Healing-Phase Diet— Weight Loss: The Allergy and Asthma Cure Step Five

Since weight loss usually involves eliminating certain foods, I thought it would be a change if we could devise a program that allowed certain foods rather than eliminated them. If you are interested in losing weight, you need to commit this chapter to memory. If you do not want to lose weight or don't need to, then please skip ahead to chapter 10. The rules in this chapter apply only to those who desire to be thinner.

If any of you are familiar with my second book, *Thin For Good,* you know that I have a keen interest in weight loss. I was the associate medical director of the Atkins Center in New York City and learned firsthand everything there is to know about low-carbohydrate dieting. However, I did see major improvements that could be made in Dr. Atkins' program. In *Thin For Good* I discuss the important difference between diets that should be followed by women and those that should be followed by men. There is a reason why men tend to lose weight faster than women. There can be no one diet that is right for everyone. I also think that it is crucial to the success of any program to incorporate one's mind into the process. It makes weight loss much easier and healthier.

I don't have room to make those distinctions here because this book is not primarily about weight loss. It is about something much more serious and debilitating—the inability to breathe, and how to correct that. If you choose to lose weight in the process, I congratulate you for that, and I certainly want to encourage it. As I have said before, studies show that weight loss can make you breathe easier. Anything you can do to help this process is going to be beneficial in the long run. As long as you are going through this program, you may as well lose weight along the way. It involves only a few more things to do.

Consider this headline from a recent medical newspaper: "Obesity Causes Asthma." How's that for being blunt? It was always assumed that those who had asthma became overweight because of their difficulty breathing. Now, according to Dr. Weiss, professor of medicine at the Channing Laboratory at Brigham and Women's Hospital in Boston, new-onset asthma is directly related to body mass index. For those with a BMI over 30, the risk of asthma is three times higher than for lean individuals. The same pattern held true for weight gain and asthma in children in the population-based Six Cities Study. Children as young as six years old and in the highest quintile of BMI had three times the risk of asthma as did those in the lowest quintile. If you are reading this book for your child, please follow the weight loss diet outlined in my book *Feed Your Kids Well*, coupled with the yeast restriction in the healing phase of this diet program. Don't put your child on a diet meant for adults. Children have different metabolic and nutritional requirements.

Now I will outline the additional things you need to remember to drop those unwanted pounds. Remember, you must also follow the advice offered in chapter 12 about yeast restrictions. If you think you can add these limitations to your diet, please do so. If you think it may be too limiting, please switch back to following the program outlined in chapter 12 only. Once you are able to breathe well again, and are excited about the program, you can always go back to this chapter. Or if you are a purist and want to know how I really feel about weight loss, you can always refer to *Thin For Good*. Until then, let's make this cure as successful as it can be.

Size Matters

This is a point that is often on people's minds, and no matter what you hear or read, size usually does matter, and with food there is no exception. This is the part of the cure where I discuss portions. I know that most other low-carbohydrate advocates would have you believe that portions don't matter—only carbohydrate grams do. That may be true for certain people, but not for the majority. Also, I am interested in teaching you how to eat for the rest of your life, not just until you lose enough weight to fit into a certain dress. No matter what else you may have read, portions are important, not only in weight loss, but also in keeping the weight off.

Although I am not that big an advocate for counting things, I believe that to begin a new lifestyle eating program, you are going to have to become aware of how much you should eat and how much you may have been eating. The portions I recommend are rather generous, and are certainly enough to satisfy almost anyone's hunger. But, overweight people don't eat because they are hungry or until they are full. That is something that I am going to try to help you change. The only way we can do that is to become aware of portions.

The suggestions I am going to make for portions are not hard-and-fast rules. They are made to give you an idea of what constitutes an appropriate-size portion. Don't think you can't be on the weight-loss component of the cure simply because you don't want to be bothered with portions. They are meant to serve as guidelines not absolutes. The biggest lesson I have learned as a former overweight person is that I can't eat everything I may want at one sitting. I now accept that, but it wasn't easy, and it still bothers me to this day.

What Can I Eat?

If you can't follow the portion controls I am going to list, you nevertheless should ensure that your diet is 65 percent protein and 35 percent complex carbohydrates. Getting that ratio is easy. Just look at your plate: about two-thirds of it should be protein. This must be done at each meal—no carbohydrate loading at one meal and protein the rest of the day. This diet is a metabolic one, and if you deviate from the 65/35 rule, even at one meal, you run the risk of messing up your metabolism for about three days. Therefore, if you cheat twice per week, you have essentially not been dieting. In this section of the diet you should focus not only on what you eat, but also on the amounts that you eat, if you can.

The suggestions in this section should be followed for about three months, or even longer if you have more weight to lose. If you have only a few pounds to lose, you may want to switch to the suggestions in chapter 8 before three months have elapsed. If you have more weight to lose by the end of the first three months, you can go off the yeast restrictions from chapter 8 but still follow the weight-loss suggestions here. I will explain how to make the transition from one phase to the next in chapter 10.

Proteins

These are going to be the main focus of your diet for the next three months or beyond, depending on the amount of weight you have to lose. Get comfortable with them, and also try to follow the extra health suggestions I made in chapter 8. It will only make you that much healthier without that much more effort. You are going to be less hungry on this diet than you have ever been before. Eating proteins without eating sugar and simple carbohydrates will help to decrease inflammation, your appetite will be normalized, you will have more energy, and your food cravings will disappear. For the entire protein category (except for eggs, which I count separately), I suggest that you keep the total daily amount to less than 24 to 30 ounces per day. If you are a man, lean toward the higher amount; if a woman, lean toward the lower amount. I will suggest amounts in each category of protein. Obviously, if you are eating only one category of protein, you may eat more than what is suggested as long as your total daily amount doesn't exceed the total allowable ounces for the day. This precludes that you are going to follow my portion control suggestion at all. Remember, it is only a suggestion and will not change the integrity of the diet if you do not follow it in the protein categories. All other portions in all other categories should be strictly adhered to.

Red Meats

All red meats are permissible in the weight-loss add-on section of the healing phase. This includes beef, veal, lamb, pork, rabbit, venison, and other game animals. I recommend that you limit your consumption of red meat to about 6 to 8 ounces per day. This is roughly the amount of meat that would fit into your hand. To help me keep within this guideline, I will buy meats in 8-ounce or 1-pound packages and divide them in two immediately, before cooking them. If you don't cook it, you won't eat it. If you are overweight, you have to start thinking of ways to help break your pattern of overeating—no matter how stupid or impractical you may think the suggestion is.

Fish

This is an excellent choice in the protein category and I recommend that you try to consume most of your protein from fish. I suggest that you eat up to 12 to 14 ounces of this very healthy source of protein per day. There are many health benefits, especially to those with allergies and/or asthma, if you consume the majority of your protein from this category. Permissible fish include but are not limited to sole, flounder, cod, tuna, swordfish, salmon, trout, mahi-mahi, tilapia, catfish, herring, pompano, bluefish, and bass. Permissible shellfish include but are not limited to oysters, crab, lobster, mussels, clams, abalone, squid, conch, shrimp, and scallops.

Poultry

All poultry is permissible on this program, including but not limited to duck, chicken, turkey, Cornish hens, pheasant, quail, and guinea hen. I suggest that you limit this category of proteins to 6 to 8 ounces per day. I also suggest that you try to limit the amount of dark meat in favor of lighter meat, as the latter has less fat.

Eggs

I think that these are a very healthy source of protein. They are included separately, and I recommend that you consume no more than 4 eggs per day. There is absolutely no link between your blood cholesterol level and the amount of eggs you consume. That has been proven wrong, so eat these to your heart's content, and I mean that literally. Lecithin, which has been shown to lower cholesterol, is in the egg yolk, so eat the yolk with the white.

Cheese

No cheese is permitted in this section of the diet due to the yeast limitations.

Complex Carbohydrates

This is a very large category of food and you must learn to think of carbohydrates as being more than bread or pasta. This category also includes things such as vegetables, fruits, and complex grain products. Complex carbohydrates are the only permissible ones in this phase of the diet program. Here is what you may choose from:

Vegetables

This group is divided into several subgroups, depending on the carbohydrate content of the vegetable.

The lowest-carbohydrate group consists of those that are less than 10 percent carbohydrate; they are generally considered the salad vegetables. This includes the green leafy lettuces and some minor additions such as iceberg, romaine, Boston, and Bibb lettuces; escarole, kale, beet greens, Swiss chard, collard greens, dandelions, radicchio, parsley, spinach, mustard greens, endive, arugula, and bok choy; fennel, celery, radishes, peppers, bean sprouts, and cucumbers also are in this section. This list is certainly not exhaustive but should give you a good representation of what is to be included in this group. You may eat these raw, frozen, cooked, or fresh. Try to eat the darker leaves, as these contain the most nutrients. Five cups per day of loosely packed greens are recommended as a maximum.

The second subgroup consists of those vegetables that are 10 to 25 percent carbohydrate. This list is the longest and contains most vegetables if they are not listed in the other two categories. These include broccoli, cauliflower, turnips, eggplant, asparagus, snow pea pods, cabbage (remember, this is not a salad vegetable), Brussels sprouts, scallions, leeks, onions, water chestnuts, zucchini, okra, artichoke hearts, string beans, and shallots. Again, these may be eaten raw, frozen, cooked, canned, or fresh. However, the maximum amount of these vegetables that you may consume in a day is $^3/_4$ cup cooked.

The third subgroup of vegetables are those highest in carbohydrates. The ones that may be eaten from this include parsnips; butternut, buttercup, or acorn squash; sweet potatoes; celery roots; artichokes; and ethnic root vegetables such as jicama, breadfruit, christophene, cassava, and plantains. Probably many other ethnic vegetables also belong in this category; for simplicity, assume that they do. These may be eaten fresh, canned, raw, frozen, or cooked. These are limited to a maximum of $1/4$ cup, cooked, once per week.

Forbidden Vegetables

During a weight loss phase, there are some vegetables you should avoid. These include tomatoes (really a fruit), white potatoes (the second most consumed vegetable in the United States), beets, peas (really a legume), carrots (too high in sugar), and corn (really more of a starch).

Grains

Any grain that you eat during the healing phase of the diet must be yeast-free. They must also be complex grains. I have taught you how to choose complex grains, so let's review.

1. Always look for the word "whole" in the ingredients list. It is not enough to say it elsewhere on the packaging.
2. Try grains you may not be familiar with, such as spelt, quinoa, amaranth, and teff.
3. Crackers are simple carbohydrates.
4. Regular pasta, artichoke or otherwise, is a simple grain and is to be avoided.
5. Breads, should you choose to eat them, must say "yeast-free" on the label.
6. Avoid any food that says it is enriched.

Whole Grains

This category of food includes brown rice (short, medium, or long grain, not wild), cracked wheat, bulgar wheat, millet, oats, barley (kasha), kamut, soy flour, milo, corn, quinoa, amaranth, spelt, and teff. These may be eaten as a cereal (hot or cold) or a side dish, and also can be used as flours for browning or thickening in recipes.

Breads

This category includes any bread that says it is yeast-free. These are becoming more and more readily available, even in regular supermarkets, so don't fear them. This may include but is not limited to sourdough (not all sourdough is yeast-free, so check the label), rye (again, not all rye is yeast-free), essene, spelt, kamut, and ezekiel. Breads may be eaten up to 1 slice per week.

Cereals

There are many cereals in this category, and most of them are yeast-free. You just have to be certain they do not contain sugar. Examples include wheat, oatmeal (not instant); brown rice, mixed whole grain; millet, corn, rice, wheat, and quinoa; and kasha. Even cereals that pretend to be healthy can be filled with sugar, so check accordingly. Carbohydrates per serving don't matter as much as grams of sugar included in the serving. Look for those cereals that have 0 to 2 grams of sugar per serving. You may ignore the carbohydrate count.

Pasta

There are healthy pasta choices you can make too. Any pasta that says it is enriched should be avoided. Healthy examples of this category include: udon (pasta made from whole wheat); soba (pasta made from buckwheat); and pasta made from corn, brown rice, spelt, quinoa, kamut, and soy. These should be cooked al dente (or somewhat hard) so they don't get mushy. In this way, they will taste more like regular pasta.

Serving Sizes

For all the grains except the breads, the suggested serving size is $1/_2$ cup, cooked, once per week, as a group. Therefore you can eat only one of this group—pasta, bread, cereals, and whole grains once per week, not each one once per week. I recommend that you do not eat all the once-per-week foods on the same day. Try to spread them out throughout the week. Not only will you lose weight quicker, but also you always will have a good carbohydrate to look forward to.

Legumes

The legumes that may be consumed include but are not limited to lentils, kidney beans, black beans, lima beans, fava beans, black-eyed peas, navy beans, and peanuts. These are allowed up to $1/_2$ cup, cooked, once per week. Again, these should not be eaten on the same day as the other once-per-week foods so that your body maintains the correct metabolic balance. For peanuts, these should be 1 ounce per day maximum, about 10 peanuts.

Nuts and Seeds

The nuts and seeds you may eat include but are not limited to pecans, walnuts, almonds, Brazil nuts, filberts, pumpkin seeds, sunflower seeds, macadamia nuts, and hazelnuts. These may be consumed up to 2 ounces per day, which is roughly 20 nuts. Try not to consume these all at once. Nuts and seeds can be very addictive because they taste so good. If you eat too many, your weight loss will slow down or not occur at all; a few will satisfy your hunger quite easily. Buy them in individual 1-ounce packages or predivide them into your suggested serving before you are hungry. It will help you stay within your limit more easily.

Nuts that are not permitted in this category include pistachios and peanuts (which are legumes). Pistachios should not be eaten if you want to lose weight.

Or

Nut butters are also in this category. These include peanut, almond, walnut, and macadamia nut butter. The limit should be 2 tablespoons per day. Eat only nut butters that are all-natural and contain nothing but the nuts. If the butter separates, then you know it is natural and contains no sugar. Sugar prevents commercial nut butters from separating.

Extras

This category includes olives, allowable up to 4 per day, and avocados, allowable up to $1/_2$ per day.

Protein Bars/Shakes

This category includes protein bars, shakes, chocolates, and other low-carbohydrate grain products such as bagels and muffins. The limits I suggest for these products are:

Protein Bars

These are allowable up to 1 per day; they are only to be used as a meal replacement, not as a snack.

Or

Protein Shakes

These are allowable up to 1 shake per day, to be used as a meal replacement, not as a snack. These tend to make a great breakfast for those who tire of eggs. People who are sensitive or allergic to milk should avoid these, since most of them are made from whey protein.

As a reminder, the bars and the shakes are an either/or proposition. You cannot have both of them on the same day. Choose wisely.

High-Protein Chocolate Bars

While these certainly taste delicious, I recommend that you save these for one serving once per week, as a treat. Please pay strict attention to serving size, as the serving size for these products is usually much less than one bar. Don't be fooled.

High-Protein Grain Products

Be very suspicious of these products. I suggest you avoid them completely in the weight-loss healing phase of the program.

Condiments/Butter/Oils

Please check that the condiments you use do not contain sugar. Most seasoning mixes contain sugar and should be avoided. Most straight spices, except curry powder, usually do not contain sugar and should be all right to use. Catsup and margarine are not allowed.

Spices

Just make sure they do not contain MSG. They can be used in unlimited amounts.

Butter/Ghee

This is allowable up to 3 tablespoons per day.

Macadamia Nut Oil

This is the preferred oil and is allowed in unlimited quantities. Olive oil is the second choice oil and is also allowed in unlimited quantities. Almost all oils contain the same amount of calories despite what is used to make the oil.

Mayonnaise/Mustard

You may use this up to 3 tablespoons per day.

Lemon/Lime Juice

This is allowable up to 4 teaspoons per day.

Beverages

Water

This is the only beverage I recommend. You may drink it sparkling, flat, distilled, filtered, spring, tap, or bottled. Water helps to keep us hydrated and helps our body to function properly. If you are properly hydrated, you can increase the functioning of your metabolism by up to 5 percent. It will be like exercising, only without the effort.

The proper amount of water that you need to drink is easily determined. As a rough estimate, simply divide your body weight in half and drink that many ounces each day. For example, if you weigh 150 pounds, you would need to drink about 75 ounces of water daily to keep your metabolism at optimum functioning. For every cup of caffeinated beverage, you must drink 2 cups of additional water. For every 45 minutes of strenuous exercise, you should increase your water consumption by 16 ounces.

I know that this is a lot of water, but it is how much your body needs to do its job. If you are drinking significantly less than I recommend, try increasing the amount of water you drink each day slowly until you reach the correct amount. You will start urinating more, but that will slowly start to adjust, and return to normal. Keep up the drinking, though; it is important for your body and for your weight loss.

Soda

Only diet soda is permitted in the weight-loss portion of the diet. I usually don't recommend that you drink this at all, but if you must, then try to limit it to 24 ounces per day. The aspartame in the diet soda may set up a blood sugar reaction, and you may get hungrier just because you drank soda. The same holds true for any artificially sweetened drink. The more aspartame, the sweeter it is, and the more your body will think it is sugar. Please be wary of this and try to avoid it. I have had many patients lose extra weight simply by eliminating diet drinks from their diet.

Coffee/Tea

The only beverage I recommend from this category is herbal tea; in fact, it can take the place of some of the water I recommend. However, drinking other teas or coffee will not upset your weight loss; I just think that herbal teas are healthier. Please try to limit your consumption of caffeinated beverages (tea usually has more caffeine than coffee, including diet iced tea beverages) to 2 cups per day. Because of the effect that caffeine can have on cortisol levels in the body and ultimately on blood sugar, I try to ask people to refrain completely. If you are going to give up caffeine cold turkey, you will probably get a headache for the first three days as your body gives up its addiction, so don't be surprised and try to stick with it.

Milk

This is not suggested in the weight-loss part of the diet. This applies to all types of milk. Milk has a lot of sugar and must be avoided—even lactose-free. Unsweetened soy and rice milk as well as goat milk also are not suggested for this part of your diet.

Heavy or light cream but not half-and-half is permissible at up to 2 tablespoons per day.

Alcohol

This is not permitted in the weight-loss section of the diet program.

Fruits

These are not suggested for the weight-loss portion of the cure.

Desserts

The only permissible commercially available dessert is diet gelatin. However, please feel free to be creative, given the recommendations and the list of acceptable ingredients. If you come up with something really good, please let me know so I may include it in my next book. My address and phone number are in chapter 15, "A Resource Guide."

As you can see, many food choices are available for the person who wants to take the cure and lose weight at the same time. There are not really that many differences, but enough to create weight loss. I really want you to be comfortable doing the diet, getting thinner, but most importantly, getting healthier. If you feel that the weight-loss diet will be too restrictive, even though you need to lose weight, don't do it. Please don't feel compelled to try to lose weight and breathe better at the same time. Don't set yourself up for failure. The most important thing to me is that you feel better, stay with the program, and give it the chance it deserves to make you healthier. If you can only follow the diet outlined in chapter 8, then do that and don't feel guilty about it. Let's just be successful at breathing better. Weight loss can wait for a while if it must.

The Allergy and Asthma Cure
Step Five: Review

1. Follow the guidelines in this chapter only if you desire to lose weight.
2. Have your food sensitivity list handy, and immediately cross off anything in this chapter that may not be permissible for you, according to your list.

3. Follow the rules for permitted foods and foods to be avoided from the yeast-free diet in chapter 8.
4. Add the rules in this chapter to your program.
5. Each meal should contain about 65 percent protein and 35 percent complex carbohydrates. This is basically $2/3$ protein and $1/3$ complex carbohydrates.
6. Protein is essentially unlimited but should be restricted to 24 to 30 ounces a day for better health.
7. Low-carbohydrate vegetables are limited to 5 cups per day.
8. Medium-carbohydrate vegetables are limited to $3/4$ cup, cooked, per day.
9. Higher-carbohydrate vegetables are limited to $1/4$ cup, cooked, once per week.
10. Whole grains, cereals, and pastas may be eaten up to $1/2$ cup, cooked, once per week, *or*
11. Yeast-free breads may be consumed up to 1 slice per week.
12. Permissible legumes may be consumed up to $1/2$ cup, cooked, once per week.
13. The once-per-week categories of food should not be eaten on the same day.
14. Permissible nuts are allowed up to 2 ounces or 2 tablespoons of nut butter per day.
15. Water should be consumed up to roughly half your body weight in pounds in ounces per day.
16. Limit high-protein bars/shakes to 1 serving of either, not both, per day; use them as meal replacements, not snacks.
17. Avoid high-protein grain products.
18. Limit high-protein candy to once per week.
19. Alcohol is not permitted.
20. Fruit or fruit juice is not permitted.
21. Milk is not permitted, but 2 tablespoons of heavy or light cream per day are.
22. Don't forget to keep your symptom questionnaire.

10

Breathing Better:
The Allergy and
Asthma Cure Step Six

By the time you get to this phase of the diet, you should be breathing better and relying much less on your medications. Review your symptom questionnaire. I am confident that your symptoms are markedly less than when you started the cure.

You are now at the most important part of the program. Most diet books can get you to lose weight. I want to make sure that you keep the weight off, and if you didn't need or want to lose weight, I want to make sure that you continue to breathe better for the rest of your life. We are in this for the long haul. Now that you have gone without certain things for three months, those things are probably far less important to you than they were when we started. Now I am going to teach you how to reintroduce certain foods into your diet that you may be missing or need back. There are certain foods I want you to avoid for the most part for the rest of your life. One would be sugar. This is not to say that you should never eat sugar or simple carbohydrates again. I would never suggest that because you would throw this book away and laugh at me. However, once patients begin to breathe better and don't need their medications, some foods that they used to eat become much less important, and they don't want them back. They just want to continue to breathe well.

Jeff, a forty-seven-year-old man, was very skeptical when he first came to see me. He only came because I had helped one of his friends so much that he had to see for himself if this was too good to be true. I tested him and started him on the program. I had never met a more skeptical patient. I was beginning to wonder why he was in my office or if I was ever going to see him again. He thought he would never be able to stay on the program, as I asked him to give up all of his favorite foods. He fought with me through the entire three months, but was diligent in following the recommended guidelines. He slowly improved each time I saw him until the last visit on the program, when he told me he had not needed his medications for the past three weeks—the only time in his life he could remember saying that.

I then congratulated him on staying with the program and told him we could now begin to allow him to have more foods. He looked at me incredulously and said, "Why would I ever want to do that? I'm breathing better than I ever have, am not using any medication, and I feel great. I don't ever want to go back to feeling the way I did." I figured he was only human, so I explained the breathing-better phase of the diet to him just in case. Three years later, he is still breathing well, and is medication-free. He has started to introduce new foods into his diet in the past year and has had no setbacks.

What Do I Do Now?

In case you are one of the few who want more food, this is the place to start. Whatever you do, do not think this is the end. "I've lasted three months and my 'diet' is over. I can now go back to eating the way I did before." That is the wrong attitude to have. If the way you ate before was successful, then you would not have been the mess you were. There are certain things you can do to ensure that you can eat the largest variety of foods while still maintaining the benefits of the cure. This will be a slow process, but it is worth doing to continue the success you have had.

There are three parts to the breathing-better phase of the diet. Each part is for a different healing phase dieter. Part A should be followed by the person who was on the non-weight-loss section of the healing-phase diet (chapter 8 only). Part B should be followed by those who incorporated the weight-loss add-ons (chapter 9) to their program and still have more weight to lose. Part C should be used by the healing-phase dieter who started on the weight-loss program (chapter 9) and who does not wish or need to lose any more weight. Therefore you need to follow only one of these parts, depending on where you started the cure.

Here are the general guidelines:

1. Every week, you will be adding new foods.
2. The types of foods you add will be determined by you according to the guidelines I set up. You will be designing your own breathing-better transition.
3. Continue to maintain and monitor your symptom questionnaire as you begin to reintroduce new foods. This is the only way you are going to be able to tell if anything is giving you a problem.

Part A: Breathing Better without Needing to Lose Weight

This is where you should be going if you had no weight to lose and/or simply followed the healing-phase diet. This transition should last about sixteen weeks. By now you will have learned an entirely new way of eating. Another four months should serve to reinforce this new behavioral pattern. The longer you can give your body to heal, the better off you are going to be in the long run. New habits take a long time to master. You are probably never going to return to your old ways of eating, so let's continue to learn new ways.

Week 1

I generally ask my patients which foods they are missing most and which they would like back. Since I can't be there to tell you whether it is an acceptable Week 1 food, I am going to give you guidelines of the foods from which I think you should choose. This is the simplest week, so simply choose any food from your food sensitivity list that was in the orange category or the 2+ category. These were your least sensitive foods. You may begin to have this food twice per week for the next week. Choose another food from the same list; you may have that twice per week in the same week, but not on the same day as the other one. For example, if you choose garlic and chicken, you may have garlic on, say, Monday and Thursday, and chicken on Tuesday and Friday.

Week 2

> Orange/2+ food sensitivities: The foods from last week may now be tried every day if you wish. Choose several more and incorporate those twice per week, but not on the same day.

Week 3

Gradually begin to get all of your least-sensitive foods back into your diet. If they are on the list and you never ate them, you don't need to start now. If you have reintroduced all that is on the minor list by now, then begin to reintroduce the red/3+ and higher category of foods.

> Orange/2+ food sensitivities: Reintroduce anything that you already haven't, according to the same schedule outlined above.

> Red/3+ or higher food sensitivities: Reintroduce two of these foods twice per week, again, not on the same day.

Note: If you have a tremendous number of food sensitivities, you may have to broaden this over the first eight weeks. Don't try to rush the process. If you have many minor food sensitivities, it may take you to week 8 before you start the red/3+ category. There are no hard-and-fast rules here. The idea is to slowly reintroduce foods that you were sensitive to over a long period of time. This helps to determine if you are still sensitive to one or if you are sensitive to a combination of the foods. You shouldn't be by this time in the cure, but I want you to be aware that you may be, and to take action accordingly. If you find your symptoms getting worse, then stop those foods and don't try them again until the end of the last week of the transition phase. We have to work together on this because the reintroduction of the food sensitivities is the hardest part of this program.

Week 4

This is the first week where we are going to introduce the foods that contain yeast or that feed yeast. I usually ask the patient which category he or she wishes to start with. I am going to decide this for you to help make this transition period easier to follow.

Orange/2+ food sensitivities: Continue to add more of these to your diet, eliminating any you still think may be causing problems.

Red/3+ or higher food sensitivities: Continue to introduce two more of these into your diet twice per week, and increase the amount of time you are eating the ones from the previous week.

Cheese: Only soft cheese is permitted at this time. Try adding 2 ounces of cream, cottage, ricotta, pot, or farmer's cheese twice per week.

Week 5

Orange/2+ food sensitivities: Continue to reintroduce these into your diet at the rate of one or two twice per week. The ones from the previous weeks can be eaten throughout the week.

Red/3+ or higher food sensitivities: Continue to reintroduce these into your diet one or two twice per week. The ones from the previous weeks can be eaten throughout the week.

Cheese: The soft cheese that you introduced last week can now be eaten 3 times per week.

Vinegar: This can be introduced up to 2 tablespoons twice per week.

Fermented foods: Two different ones can be reintroduced twice per week, but not on the same days.

Week 6

Orange/2+ food sensitivities: Continue the slow process of reintroducing these foods as described above.

Red/3+ or higher food sensitivities: Continue the slow process of reintroducing these foods as described above.

Cheese: The soft cheeses can now be eaten up to 3 ounces per day every day of the week.

Vinegar: This can now be eaten up to 2 tablespoons per day.

Fermented foods: These can now be eaten up to every day. A different one should be eaten each day.

Edible fungi: These are mushrooms, which can be eaten $1/2$ cup, cooked, twice per week.

Week 7

Orange/2+ food sensitivities: Unless you have a very long list, you should have already reintroduced all of these into your diet. If not, then continue at a slow rate of reintroduction.

Red/3+ food sensitivities: This also includes any higher sensitivity that your food sensitivity test may have registered. Continue the slow process with these foods.

Cheese: Continue with the soft cheeses only.

Vinegar: Continue with the 2 tablespoons per day. Any condiment that you were avoiding because it had vinegar in it may now be reintroduced. Any food that you were avoiding because it contained vinegar, such as bottled salad dressings (as long as it doesn't have sugar), may be added. Pickles may now be reintroduced twice per week.

Fermented foods: Continue at the same rate of introduction of new ones.

Edible fungi: These may now be eaten $1/2$ cup, cooked, three times per week.

Smoked meats or fish: These may now be added up to 2 ounces twice per week.

Week 8

Orange/2+ food sensitivities: Continue the slow reintroduction process.

Red/3+ or higher food sensitivities: Continue the slow reintroduction process.

Cheese: Continue with the soft cheeses only.

Vinegar: Continue with the current amount of vinegar.

Fermented foods: Continue with the same amount of these foods.

Edible fungi: These may now be consumed at $1/2$ cup, cooked, every day.

Smoked meats or fish: Continue with 2 ounces twice per week.

Third subgroup of vegetables: These may now be eaten at 1 cup, cooked, every day.

Week 9

Do not add anything additional to your diet during this week. This will allow your body to catch up metabolically and also will allow you to notice any subtle negative changes that may have occurred during this period of reintroduction.

Week 10

Orange/2+ food sensitivities: Continue the slow reintroduction process.

Red/3+ or higher food sensitivities: Continue the slow reintroduction process.

Cheese: Continue to eat the soft cheeses. You may now add 2 ounces of hard cheese every day that is not moldy or aged, such as mozzarella, Monterey Jack, Muenster, etc.

Vinegar: This continues at the same rate as before.

Fermented foods: This continues as before.

Edible fungi: This continues at the same amount as before.

Smoked meats/fish: This continues at the same amount as before.

Third subgroup of vegetables: This continues at the same amount as before.

Fruits: I consider some fruits to have better nutritional value than others, and I have divided these into four subgroups. The first subgroup contains all the melons and the berries. This includes but is not limited to blueberries, strawberries, raspberries, watermelon, cantaloupes, and honeydew. The second subgroup consists of grapefruit, peaches, plums, pears, and nectarines. The third subgroup comprises apples, kiwis, and oranges. The fourth subgroup includes all the tropical fruits such as bananas, mangoes, papayas, and guavas. If there is a fruit I did not mention in any of these categories and it is *not* tropical, then it goes into the third category. That is a general rule of thumb and one that will work to your advantage.

The first subgroup of fruits is now permissible up to $1/2$ cup twice per week.

Week 11

Orange/2+ food sensitivities: Continue to slowly reintroduce these.

Red/3+ or higher food sensitivities: Continue to slowly reintroduce these.

Cheese: The amounts of these remain the same.

Vinegar: This remains the same.

Fermented foods: These remain the same.

Edible fungi: These remain the same.

Smoked meats/fish: You may now have these up to 4 ounces twice per week.

Third subgroup of vegetables: These remain the same.

Fruits: These remain the same.

Alcohol: In this category, I also believe there are subgroups that should be noted. The first subgroup is the brown liquors. This includes scotch, bourbon, whiskey, and rye. The second subgroup comprises all the white liquors such as vodka and gin, but not rum and cachaça. The third subgroup includes rum, cachaça, beer, and wine. You are now allowed to have 2 ounces from *either* the first or the second subgroup.

Legumes: You may now have this category of food up to 1 cup, cooked, 4 times per week.

Week 12

Orange/2+ food sensitivities: Continue to slowly reintroduce these.

Red/3+ or higher food sensitivities: Continue to slowly reintroduce these.

Cheese: This remains the same.

Vinegar: This remains the same.

Fermented foods: These remain the same.

Edible fungi: These remain the same.

Smoked meats/fish: These remain the same.

Third subgroup of vegetables: These remain the same.

Fruits: These remain the same.

Alcohol: This remains the same.

Legumes: These remain the same.

Complex grains: These remain the same.

This week is similar to week 9, whereby you have to give your body a chance to rest and assimilate all the new foods it is now eating. Food sensitivities can sometimes take two weeks before becoming a problem, and since this week represents the third month, it is possible to see some reactions creep in at this point. Pay careful attention to your symptom questionnaire, and do not introduce any other foods except as indicated.

Week 13

Orange/2+ food sensitivities: Continue with the slow reintroduction process.

Red/3+ or higher food sensitivities: Continue with the slow reintroduction process.

Cheese: You may now have up to 4 ounces per day of the hard cheeses. The soft cheeses remain the same.

Vinegar: This remains the same.

Fermented foods: These remain the same.

Edible fungi: These remain the same.

Smoked meats/fish: You may now have up to 4 ounces three times per week.

Third subgroup of vegetables: These remain the same.

Fruits: You may now have $1/2$ cup of the first subgroup every day.

Alcohol: This remains the same.

Legumes: These remain the same.

Complex grains: You may now have 1 cup, cooked, four times per week.

Week 14

Orange/2+ food sensitivities: Continue with the reintroduction process.

Red/3+ or higher food sensitivities: Continue with the reintroduction process.

Cheese: Continue with the same amounts.

Vinegar: This remains the same.

Fermented foods: These remain the same.

Edible fungi: These remain the same.

Smoked meats/fish: You may now have these every day.

Third subgroup of vegetables: These remain the same.

Fruits: You may now have the second subgroup of fruit $1/2$ cup twice per week but not on the same days as the first subgroup.

Alcohol: This remains the same.

Legumes: You may now have this group every day.

Complex grains: You may now have 1 cup, cooked, up to five times per week.

Tomatoes/peas/carrots/potatoes: You may now have these up to $1/2$ cup, cooked, twice per week. This is the last of the food groups that you haven't been eating up to now.

Week 15

Everything remains the same except:

Cheese: You may now have the moldy, aged cheeses such as blue, Roquefort, and Parmesan up to 2 ounces twice per week.

Fruits: You may now have the second subgroup up to five times per week.

Week 16

Everything remains the same except:

Cheese: You may now have the older cheeses from last week up to five times per week.

Fruits: You may now have the third subgroup of fruits $1/_2$ cup twice per week.

Complex grains: These may now be eaten up to 1 cup, cooked, every day.

Tomatoes/peas/carrots/potatoes: You may now enjoy these up to $1/_2$ cup, cooked, five times per week.

Over time, if you have followed this plan, you will have incorporated virtually everything back into your diet that is healthy. The subgroups of foods I did not mention, such as the third subgroup of alcohol or the fourth subgroup of fruits, are foods that I place in the same category as sugar and simple carbohydrates. I think you should always avoid them; if you can't, then leave them for special occasions or have them very rarely, less than once per month.

Since I know you are feeling so much better, by now you are willing to go through this lengthy process. Because the program is individualized, it is likely that you may not get through the entire sixteen weeks. There may be foods that you cannot reintroduce into your diet. If that is the case, then just wait longer and try once per month or less until you get to a happy medium between what you want to eat and what your body says you can. By the end of this cure, you are going to be so attuned to your body's needs that you will know how far you can push the envelope.

Part B: Breathing Better and Losing Weight

This is where you should continue if you have lost weight in the healing phase and wish to lose more. There will be different things you need to do than in part A. Once you have followed these steps and have gotten to the point where you don't need or want to lose any more weight, simply follow part C. The amount of time you continue to spend in this phase will be determined by how much weight you want to lose. This phase could even take a year or more. Most people will lose an average of 2 pounds per week. This is a very healthy weight loss, and one that can easily be maintained. Therefore, if you have 100 pounds to lose, you may be on this phase of the diet for a year. It all depends on your needs. However, the transition to your breathing-better phase should not take more than six weeks.

You must refer to your food sensitivity lists again at this point. We are going to begin to reintroduce foods that, depending on your list, may take longer than the six weeks. You should start reintroducing the foods you were least sensitive to. Depending on the test your doctor ordered, this will be in the orange/2 + category. The red/3 + or higher food sensitivities also will be reintroduced, but later in the program. This will be strictly determined by you and the reactions you are getting. You probably will not get any reactions, but you should be prepared to stop eating the food again if you find your symptoms getting worse or your need for medication increasing. Keep your symptom questionnaire close at hand and continue to fill it out through this transition phase B. Everyone will have a slightly individual reaction to the reintroduction of foods, and since I will not be there to help you, you are going to have to judge whether you need to eliminate a certain food or keep it in your program.

Week 1

Orange/2 + food sensitivities: Choose the foods from this category that you desire the most, as long as they stay within the weight-loss guideline of the diet. For example, if you are sensitive to cane sugar, I do not want you adding that back to your diet. Choose acceptable foods from this category and reintroduce two of them into your diet twice per week, but not on the same day.

Red/3 + or higher food sensitivities: Do not reintroduce any from this list yet.

Proteins: The amount of protein I suggest will remain the same throughout this phase of your diet.

Vegetables: The amount of vegetables I suggest will remain the same through this phase of your diet.

Complex carbohydrates: The amount of these foods will remain the same throughout this phase of your diet.

Cheese: The soft cheeses such as pot, farmer, ricotta, cream, and cottage are now allowable up to 2 ounces twice per week. These can make a great breakfast.

Week 2

Orange/2+ food sensitivities: The foods you chose last week may now be eaten every day. Choose two more foods and have them twice per week—again, not on the same day. This is the pattern you are going to be following until every minor food sensitivity you have is reintroduced into your diet. For some it may take quite a while to go through this list. You should be reintroducing only the foods permitted in the weight-loss phase of the diet.

Red/3+ or higher food sensitivities: Do not reintroduce these yet.

Proteins/vegetables/complex carbohydrates: These remain the same.

Cheese: You may now add 2 ounces of soft cheese (pot, farmer, ricotta, cream, or cottage) to your diet three times per week.

Week 3

Orange/2+ food sensitivities: Continue to slowly add these back into your diet, as described above.

Red/3+ or higher food sensitivities: The foods from this list may now be added back into your diet. Start with two foods twice per week, not eaten on the same day. The following week you are going to try to eat these more than twice per week, or you are going to add new ones from this list into your diet. This process may take some time, depending on how many foods are on this list. If you keep to this slow process, you should not have any trouble reintroducing these foods. Always refer to your symptom questionnaire, and if you notice any new problems, eat less of the food reintroduced that week, or eliminate it from your diet completely.

Proteins/vegetables/complex carbohydrates: These remain the same.

Cheese: You may now have the soft cheeses at 3 ounces three times per week. You may now reintroduce hard cheeses such as Muenster, mozzarella, Monterey Jack, etc., except for the aged, moldy varieties up to 2 ounces twice per week on the days when you are not eating the soft cheeses.

Alcohol: You may now add 1 ounce of the brown or white liquors twice per week. This includes scotch, bourbon, whiskey, gin, and vodka.

Week 4

Orange/2+ food sensitivities: Continue your present rate of reintroducing these foods.

Red/3+ or higher food sensitivities: Continue the slow rate of reintroducing these foods, in the process described above.

Proteins/vegetables/complex carbohydrates: These will remain the same.

Cheese: You may now have the soft cheeses 3 ounces per day, and the hard cheeses as above 2 ounces three times per week.

Alcohol: You may now have 1 ounce of the permitted liquors three times per week.

Fruits: You may now have the first subgroup of fruits as described in part A up to $1/2$ cup twice per week. You will recall that this group consists of all the berries and melons only.

Week 5

Orange/2+ food sensitivities: Continue with your present rate of reintroduction.

Red/3+ or higher food sensitivities: Continue with your present rate of reintroduction.

Proteins/vegetables/complex carbohydrates: These remain the same.

Cheese: You may now increase the hard cheeses to 3 ounces three times per week and leave the soft cheeses at 3 ounces every day.

Alcohol: You may now increase your limit to 2 ounces three times per week of the allowable liquors.

Fruits: This category remains the same.

Week 6

Orange/2+ food sensitivities: Continue as you have been doing.

Red/3+ or higher food sensitivities: Continue as you have been doing.

Proteins/vegetables/complex carbohydrates: These remain the same.

Cheese: Keep the soft cheeses at 3 ounces per day and increase the hard cheeses to 3 ounces per day. You may now add aged, moldy cheeses such as Roquefort, blue, or Parmesan to the hard cheese total. This is not additional, but is to be included in the total for the day. Start with these twice per week and build up as you see how well you do.

Alcohol: This remains the same.

Fruits: These remain the same.

The foods I did not mention as permitted to add should not be added to your diet at this time. Once you have lost all the weight you wish to lose, read the instructions in part C; that will help you move into the breathing-better maintenance diet program. You may not be ready for this part for a while; there is nothing wrong with that. Once a person loses weight, I believe that he or she should keep it off forever. If it takes a while to bring certain foods back on line with your diet, that's what has to occur for you to be successful. Dieting has one of the highest rates of failure, with most dieters experiencing the yo-yo syndrome. I don't want this to happen to any of the people who follow my cure, so please abide by the rules and only go to C when you are ready. Also, if you have not finished reintroducing the foods you were sensitive to, keep on going throughout part B. This is a completely individual thing, depending on how many foods you started with, so it will be different for everyone. As long as you have followed the guideline, you should be losing weight, breathing easier, and using fewer medications. Congratulations!

Summary of Foods to Eat by the End of Part B

Nothing has really changed except that I have reintroduced foods into your diet program that were eliminated because of your yeast problem. Therefore, each *meal* should still contain roughly 65 percent protein and 35 percent complex carbohydrates. If you have forgotten information regarding the following list, please refer to the full explanation in chapter 9. The following is simply meant as a quick guide to keep you on the right track.

Proteins: The amount of proteins is essentially unlimited, but I encourage patients to remain within 24 to 30 ounces per day, maximum.

Low-carbohydrate vegetables: These are limited to 5 cups per day.

Medium-carbohydrate vegetables: These are limited to $3/4$ cup, cooked, per day.

Higher-carbohydrate vegetables: These are limited to $1/4$ cup, cooked, once per week.

Whole-grain cereals/pasta and grains: These are limited to $1/2$ cup, cooked, once per week.

Or

Yeast-free breads: These are limited to 1 slice per week.

Permissible legumes: These are limited to $1/2$ cup, cooked, once per week.

Cheese: Totals of 3 ounces of soft cheeses and 3 ounces of hard cheeses are allowed each day.

Alcohol: A total of 2 ounces of the permitted liquors three times per week.

Fruits: A total of $1/2$ cup of melons or berries twice per week.

Remember that the foods recommended to be eaten only on several days per week should be eaten on different days.

Part C: Breathing Better and Maintaining Weight Loss

There are two groups of people who should be following part C. They are:

- Those who were following the weight-loss healing-phase diet found in chapter 9 and have lost all the weight they want to or are very close to their goal weight.
- People who started on the weight-loss diet in chapter 9, then followed part B, and have now achieved their desired weight.

This section of the program is going to help you transition not only from a yeast-free diet but from a weight-loss diet, too. Most people who are on a diet program like to resume their old way of eating immediately upon reaching a goal. My goal is for you to breathe better and be allergy-free for the rest of your life. That is why it is critical for you to allow your body to continue the process of healing and reducing the inflammation by sticking with this program longer. By the end of the process outlined here, you will have reintroduced most healthy foods into your diet, with the exception of sugar and simple carbohydrates—no one should be eating those. You will be healthier, breathing easier, and using less medication. You must continue to keep your symptom questionnaire so you can know immediately whether new foods you are adding may be giving you any symptoms —it will be an invaluable tool to keep this cure going for the rest of your life.

This is going to be a sixteen-week transition process to the breathing-better phase of your diet. Take your time. The foods that we are going to start with are those that were listed as your food sensitivities. By the end of the three-month healing phase, your body should be able to start incorporating the foods to which you are sensitive. Simply choose the foods you want to start with. Everyone will make different choices. I will tell you how to add them, but you must choose the foods. However, you must not add foods that are otherwise prohibited. For example, if you are allergic to cane sugar, that cannot be the first thing you add back because I recommend not eating sugar. Another example of sugar is milk. I will advise you when to reintroduce certain categories of foods into your diet. Just choose the foods that have already been allowed but that you were specifically avoiding because they were on your food sensitivity list. Don't be impatient at this point in the process. You are almost there; a few more weeks will only make the cure work longer.

Week 1

Proteins/vegetables/complex carbohydrates: These remain the same.

Orange/2+ food sensitivities: Choose two foods that you would like to reintroduce into your diet. You may have these twice per week, but not on the same day.

Week 2

Proteins/vegetables/complex carbohydrates: These remain the same.

Orange/2+ food sensitivities: The ones from last week may now be eaten every day. Choose two additional foods to add twice per week. This is the pattern you are going to follow throughout this process. Because everyone will have a different number of food sensitivities, this process will last a variable amount of weeks. For some it may take the entire sixteen weeks, or even longer. For others it will take much less time. Do it at your own pace, and keep a mindful eye on your symptom questionnaire: If any symptom gets worse and there is no other reason for it, then please stop the food immediately.

Week 3

Proteins/vegetables/complex carbohydrates: These remain the same.

Orange/2+ food sensitivities: Continue at the rate described above.

Red/3+ or higher food sensitivities: These will be added the same way as the more minor food sensitivities were. This week, add two foods you prefer into your diet twice per week, but not on the same day.

Week 4

Proteins/vegetables/complex carbohydrates: These remain the same.

Orange/2+ food sensitivities: Continue at the same rate.

Red/3+ or higher food sensitivities: You may now have the two you added last week up to every day. Choose two more from the list and try them twice per week. This is the process you will continue to follow throughout the rest of this phase until you have exhausted your list.

Cheese: You may now add cheese to your diet, but only the soft cheeses—cottage, cream, pot, farmer, or ricotta—up to 2 ounces twice per week.

Week 5

Proteins/vegetables/complex carbohydrates: These remain the same.

Orange/2+ food sensitivities: Continue to reintroduce these foods at the same rate.

Red/3+ or higher food sensitivities: Continue to reintroduce these foods at the previously described rate.

Cheese: You may now increase the soft cheeses to 2 ounces three times per week.

Alcohol: You may now have the first subgroup of alcohols, which are the brown liquors such as scotch, bourbon, whiskey, and rye; or the second subgroup of alcohols, which are the white liquors such as gin and vodka (but not rum or cachaça) up to 1 ounce twice per week. The third subgroup includes rum, cachaça, beer, and wine and is to be avoided.

Week 6

Proteins/complex carbohydrates: These remain the same.

Orange/2+ food sensitivities: Continue to reintroduce these foods.

Red/3+ or higher food sensitivities: Continue to reintroduce these foods.

Cheese: Continue with the soft cheeses, and you may now introduce hard cheeses such as mozzarella, Monterey Jack, and Muenster up to 2 ounces twice per week. Continue to avoid the aged, moldy cheeses at this time. Do not have them on the same days.

Alcohol: You may now increase the alcohol from the previous week to 1 ounce three times per week.

Second subgroup of vegetables: These may now be increased to 1 cup, cooked, per day.

Week 7

Proteins/complex carbohydrates: These remain the same.

Orange/2+ food sensitivities: Continue to reintroduce these foods at the same rate.

Red/3+ or higher food sensitivities: Continue to reintroduce these foods at the rate described above.

Cheese: The soft cheeses may now be eaten 2 ounces every day and the hard cheeses remain the same.

Alcohol: This remains the same.

Second subgroup of vegetables: These remain the same.

Third subgroup of vegetables: These may now be increased to $^1/_4$ cup, cooked, three times per week.

Edible fungi: This category includes mushrooms, which may now be eaten $^1/_2$ cup, cooked, twice per week.

Fruits: These may now be reintroduced into your diet. The first subgroup includes melons and berries. The second subgroup comprises peaches, plums, apricots, pears, and grapefruit. The third subgroup is apples, oranges, and kiwis. The fourth subgroup includes tropical fruits such as bananas, mangoes, papayas, and guavas. The first subgroup of fruits may now be added to your diet up to $^1/_2$ cup twice per week.

Week 8

Proteins: These remain the same.

Orange/2+ food sensitivities: Continue to reintroduce these foods as described above.

Red/3+ or higher food sensitivities: Continue to reintroduce these foods as described above.

Cheese: The soft cheeses remain the same; the hard cheeses you have previously been eating may now be increased to 2 ounces three times per week.

Alcohol: This remains the same.

Second subgroup of vegetables: These remain the same.

Third subgroup of vegetables: These remain the same.

Edible fungi: These remain the same.

Vinegar: This can now be reintroduced to your diet up to 2 tablespoons three times per week.

Complex grains/pasta: These can now be increased to $^1/_2$ cup, cooked, three times per week or 1 slice of yeast-free bread three times per week.

Fruits: These remain the same.

Week 9

Proteins: These remain the same.

Orange/2+ food sensitivities: Continue to reintroduce these foods as above.

Red/3+ or higher food sensitivities: Continue to reintroduce these foods as above.

Cheese: This remains the same.

Alcohol: This remains the same.

Second subgroup of vegetables: These can now be increased to $1^1/_2$ cups, cooked, per day.

Third subgroup of vegetables: These remain the same.

Edible fungi: These may now be increased to $^1/_2$ cup, cooked, five times per week.

Vinegar: This can be increased to 2 tablespoons every day.

Complex grains/pasta: These remain the same.

Fruits: The first subgroup can now be increased to $^1/_2$ cup five times per week.

Fermented foods: These can now be reintroduced into your diet. Choose two of these and eat them twice per week but not on the same day.

Week 10

Proteins: These remain the same.

Orange/2+ food sensitivities: Continue to reintroduce these foods as above.

Red/3+ or higher food sensitivities: Continue to reintroduce these foods as above.

Cheese: This remains the same.

Second subgroup of vegetables: These remain the same.

Third Subgroup of vegetables: You may now increase these to $^1/_2$ cup, cooked, three times per week.

Edible fungi: These may now be eaten up to $^1/_2$ cup, cooked, every day.

Vinegar: This remains the same.

Complex grains/pasta: These remain the same.

Fruits: These remain the same.

Fermented foods: These remain the same.

Smoked meats/fish: These can now be reintroduced to your diet up to 2 ounces twice per week.

Week 11

Proteins: These remain the same.

Orange/2+ food sensitivities: Continue to reintroduce these foods.

Red/3+ or higher food sensitivities: Continue to reintroduce these foods.

Cheese: You may now increase the amount of soft cheese you eat to 3 ounces every day, and you can increase the hard cheeses you have been eating to 3 ounces every day.

Second subgroup of vegetables: These remain the same.

Third subgroup of vegetables: These remain the same.

Edible fungi: These remain the same.

Vinegar: This remains the same.

Complex grains/pasta: These remain the same.

Fruits: You may now add the second subgroup of fruits and have those up to $1/_2$ cup on the other two days of the week.

Fermented foods: These remain the same.

Smoked meats/fish: These remain the same.

Legumes: You may now increase these to $1/_2$ cup, cooked, three times per week.

Week 12

Proteins: These remain the same.

Orange/2+ food sensitivities: Continue to reintroduce these foods.

Red/3+ or higher food sensitivities: Continue to reintroduce these foods.

Cheese: This remains the same.

Second subgroup of vegetables: These remain the same.

Third subgroup of vegetables: You may now increase these to $^1/_2$ cup, cooked, four times per week.

Edible fungi: These remain the same.

Vinegar: This remains the same.

Complex grains/pasta: These may now be increased to $^1/_2$ cup, cooked, four times per week or 1 slice of yeast-free bread four times per week.

Fruits: These remain the same.

Fermented foods: Continue to reintroduce these into your diet.

Smoked meats/fish: These may now be increased to 2 ounces four times per week.

Legumes: These remain the same.

Week 13

You should take this week off from adding any new foods. This will give your body a chance to adjust to all the new foods you have been adding. Pay close attention to your symptom questionnaire and make any necessary dietary adjustments that you see fit. If you find yourself starting to gain a little weight, either increase your amount of exercise or decrease the amount of higher-carbohydrate foods I have been allowing. This will give your body the extra time it needs to reintroduce these healthy carbohydrates into your diet. Everyone is different in the amount of carbohydrates they can add back and in the time it takes; I can only give you guidelines.

Week 14

Proteins: These remain the same.

Orange/2+ food sensitivities: Continue to reintroduce these foods.

Red/3+ or higher food sensitivities: Continue to reintroduce these foods.

Cheese: This remains the same.

Second subgroup of vegetables: These remain the same.

Third subgroup of vegetables: These may now be increased to $\frac{1}{2}$ cup, cooked, five times per week.

Edible fungi: These remain the same.

Vinegar: This remains the same.

Complex grains/pasta: These remain the same.

Fruits: These remain the same.

Fermented foods: These remain the same.

Smoked meats/fish: These remain the same.

Legumes: These may now be increased to $\frac{1}{2}$ cup, cooked, four times per week.

Week 15

Proteins: These remain the same.

Orange/2+ food sensitivities: Continue to reintroduce these foods.

Red/3+ or higher food sensitivities: Continue to reintroduce these foods.

Cheese: This remains the same, except that now you can introduce the aged or moldy cheeses such as Parmesan, aged cheddar, Roquefort, and blue cheese at 2 ounces twice per week. This is not in addition to the other cheeses, but you may substitute some of these for what you may have been eating.

Second subgroup of vegetables: These remain the same.

Third subgroup of vegetables: These remain the same.

Edible fungi: These remain the same.

Vinegar: This remains the same.

Complex grains/pasta: This remains the same.

Fruits: You may now incorporate the third subgroup of fruits into your diet at $\frac{1}{2}$ cup twice per week. This should not be in addition to the fruits you are already eating, but as a substitute for other fruits.

Fermented foods: Continue to reintroduce these.

Smoked meats/fish: These remain the same.

Legumes: These remain the same.

Forbidden vegetables: These include peas, carrots, corn, and potatoes; they may now be added to your diet at $1/2$ cup, cooked,
twice per week.

Week 16

Proteins: These remain the same.

Orange/2+ food sensitivities: Continue to reintroduce these foods.

Red/3+ or higher food sensitivities: Continue to reintroduce
these foods.

Cheese: You may now increase the amount of aged, moldy cheese
in your diet to 3 ounces five times per week. Remember, this is
not in addition to the other cheeses but as a substitute for
another type of hard cheese.

Second subgroup of vegetables: These remain the same.

Third subgroup of vegetables: These remain the same.

Edible fungi: These remain the same.

Vinegar: This remains the same.

Complex grains/pasta: You may now increase these to $1/2$ cup,
cooked, five times per week or 1 slice of yeast-free bread five
times per week. At this point you should be able to introduce
non-yeast-free bread. Try 1 slice once per week and then add 1
slice each day each week. By this time you are so used to eating yeast-free bread that you probably will not want to go back.
Whatever you do, this is not an invitation to eat a simple carbohydrate. The bread you eat must be a good whole-grain bread.

Fruits: These remain the same.

Fermented foods: These remain the same.

Smoked meats/fish: You may now increase these in your diet to 4
ounces up to every day.

Legumes: You may now increase these to $1/2$ cup, cooked, five
times per week.

Forbidden vegetables: You may now try to increase these in your
diet up to $1/2$ cup, cooked, four times per week.

There are certain foods I have not mentioned. These include the fourth subgroup of fruits and the third subgroup of alcohol. I think of these categories of food in the same way I think of sugar: Avoid them except on special occasions. I know that for fruits, this will not be hard to follow. However, many people don't want to live without beer or wine. Beer is probably one of the worst things an allergy or asthma sufferer can drink. It is a simple carbohydrate and is made by introducing yeast into the brew. Those are the two main things that I think lead to an inability to breathe well. Wine is nothing but simple sugar. It is the one food that I have the most difficulty convincing people to avoid. It can probably be had sparingly and is better than beer at least. However, in my clinical experience, many people with weight problems tend to gain weight if they reintroduce wine into their diet. Use these two products at your own risk. Just ask yourself, "Is it worth it?"

Congratulations! You have made it through the transition phase to the breathing-better segment of the cure. By this time you should have all the foods you can possibly want in your diet; have lost weight if that was your intention; be breathing significantly better; have many fewer allergy symptoms; and have reduced your reliance on pharmaceutical medications, on the advice of your physician, of course. What an accomplishment!

However, there is one more important thing to address. A good program also will require that you take some nutritional supplements. Please read on so you will know the supplements that I put my patients on to help them get rid of their allergies, breathe better, and take the cure.

The Allergy and Asthma Cure Step Six: Review

1. Maintain your symptom questionnaire and note how much better you feel and how many fewer medications you are using. Check with your doctor to make sure everything is going as well as you and I both know it is. Use this to help you determine if something you have reintroduced into your diet is troubling you. If it is, simply don't eat it, or wait a few weeks longer to reintroduce it.

2. If you were on the non-weight-loss healing phase (chapter 8), follow the guidelines in part A.
3. If you were on the weight-loss healing phase (chapter 9) and still have more weight to lose, follow the guidelines in part B.
4. Once you have lost all the weight you wish to lose, by following part B, refer to part C as to how to increase your diet even more without gaining any weight.
5. If you were on the weight-loss healing phase (chapter 9) and do not wish to lose any more weight by the end of the three months, go right to part C.
6. Continue to monitor your symptom questionnaire. If you have any additional symptoms with the reintroduction of foods, then eliminate those foods and try adding them again a few weeks later.

11

Nutritional Supplements to Treat Allergies: The Allergy and Asthma Cure Step Seven

Nutritional supplements are a critical component of the allergy and asthma cure. I rely on these harmless supplements to help my patients rid themselves of some, if not all, of their medication. Please remember that the word "supplement" means just that—a supplement to everything else I am asking you to do. You cannot jump immediately to this part of the book and expect to cure yourself of your allergies and asthma. You must follow the diet program and try to eliminate any potential allergens from your environment to the best of your ability. The programs I design for my patients are quite individualistic. Since you are not going to be my patient but must rely on using this book, I will describe several tiers of supplements I use. The first tier will be the ones I place everyone on. The next tiers will be other supplements I use in case the first tier isn't providing enough relief. The program is going to take time to work, so you must give it at least three months before thinking it is not going to work for you. I have had almost 100 percent success with the patients I treat in this manner, so there is no reason to think that you won't be part of my many success stories. When you do become another successful case, then please write to me so I can share in your happiness.

Please read this chapter whether you have allergies, asthma, sinusitis, rhinitis, or any of the skin conditions that can be helped with this program. Although this chapter is primarily aimed at the person with allergies, since these conditions are caused by the same underlying mechanism, the information in this chapter will be useful to you, too, if you suffer from them.

I am not suggesting that you ignore the advice of your regular doctor completely during this process. He or she will be invaluable in helping you to decrease your medication—something to be done only under that person's guidance. Only your regular doctor can determine if this program is right for you.

Can't I Get All the Vitamins and Minerals I Need from the Foods I Eat?

Unfortunately, you can't; otherwise, I wouldn't need to write this chapter. It is simply impossible for many reasons, the first being that our soils are mostly depleted of good minerals, and the second being that we improperly cook the foods we eat. However, I would like to mention some foods that are quite nutritious if cooked wisely.

It has been shown that most people are trying to eat more vegetables. Nearly half of us have reached the recommendations set forth by the National Cancer Institute. However, in my opinion, most of what we are eating is devoid of any health benefit. Iceberg lettuce, tomatoes, French fries, bananas, and orange juice are the top choices. Bananas, tomatoes, and orange juice have too much sugar. French fries are not that healthy for a variety of reasons, the least being that they are not really a vegetable; and iceberg lettuce has almost no nutritional value. Therefore we need supplementation.

It was reported by Dr. Adam Drewnowski and Carmen Gomez-Carneros in a recent issue of *American Journal of Clinical Nutrition* that most, if not all, of the biologically active compounds in fruits and vegetables that appear to lower the risk of cancer and heart disease are "bitter, acrid, or astringent and therefore aversive to the consumer." Plants contain unpleasant-tasting substances such as phenol, flavonoids, isoflavones, terpenes, and glucosinolates to protect them against being eaten by insects and other predators. Unfortunately, it keeps many of us away from them, too. We end up trying to disguise these tastes, and in the process, ruin the health benefits from them. That is why so many of us are turning to nutritional supplements to get the nutrition found in these healthy plant compounds.

It has been well documented that various kinds of produce may protect us from heart disease, stroke, cancer, cataracts, lung disease, diverticulosis, and possibly high blood pressure. We simply need to incorporate more of those foods into our diets to get the micronutrients that are important to our health.

Vitamins can help prevent disease, and they are the only source of certain coenzymes necessary for metabolism, the biochemical processes that support life. Certain vitamins act as antioxidants—substances that protect the body's cells from the damage caused by air pollution, chemicals, alcohol (all triggers for allergies and asthma), and the by-products of metabolism. Minerals are essential to both structure and function within the body. We have to get more of these in our diets—one way or another.

Selected Foods That Contain Vitamins

Here are some of the best foods you can eat that not only contain protein but also contain these micronutrients, which are so essential to life:

Almonds: These contain calcium, copper, vitamin E, folic acid, iron, magnesium, manganese, niacin, phosphorus, riboflavin, and zinc.

Avocados: These contain vitamins A, B_6, C, and E, copper, folic acid, magnesium, manganese, niacin, and potassium.

Broccoli: This contains vitamins A, B_6, and C, beta-carotene, folic acid, manganese, and potassium.

Pinto beans: These contain vitamin B_6, iron, folic acid, magnesium, phosphorus, and thiamin.

Spinach: This contains vitamins A, C, and E, beta-carotene, calcium, folic acid, iron, magnesium, manganese, potassium, and riboflavin.

Tuna: This contains vitamins B_6 and B_{12}, iron, magnesium, niacin, phosphorus, potassium, and omega-3 fatty acids.

Vitamins in Certain Foods

Vitamin C is in red peppers, broccoli, green peppers, Brussels sprouts, and strawberries.

Vitamin B_6 is in tuna, salmon, chicken, turkey, pork, avocados, and beef.

Folic acid is in beans, spinach, asparagus, avocados, Brussels sprouts, broccoli, and corn.

Beta-carotene is in collard greens, sweet potatoes, cantaloupes, kale, and spinach.

Potassium is in beet greens, avocados, beans, clams, and most fish.

Calcium is in peanuts, collard greens, fish skins, sardines, and salmon.

Magnesium is in almonds, hazelnuts, spinach, Swiss chard, sunflower seeds, halibut, mackerel, brown rice, tofu, beans, and avocados.

Selenium is in Brazil nuts, tuna, oysters, flounder, sole, turkey, chicken, brown rice, and eggs.

Zinc is in oysters, crab, beef, turkey, lamb, pork, almonds, beans, and chicken.

This is just a small list of healthy foods you should eat more of to get good, healthy micronutrients. Often patients will ask me if they can just eat better foods. I devised these lists to help them in their quest. Unfortunately, we have to eat so much of these foods to get the amount of nutrients we need that it becomes impractical, so nutritional supplements come into the picture and play an important role.

How to Take Nutritional Supplements

If you have never been on a nutritional supplement program, you need to be careful in how you start. Just taking a vitamin pill or two every day will not prepare you for the number of supplements I am about to recommend. Therefore, since you will be on the anticandida program *and* another program of supplements designed for your particular ailment, you need to learn how to take the supplements.

For example, if the total number of pills I recommend per day is thirty, that would roughly mean you are going to be taking ten at each meal. For the first day, I want you to take those ten and spread them out throughout the day, so you will start with three pills at each meal. Do that for a few days and then slowly increase the number of pills you take each day by one until you get to the full amount. Getting a side effect from doing this incorrectly is one of the main reasons why patients don't stay on the program. Slowly build up to the number of supplements I recommend. Some people will take longer to do this than others. That is acceptable as long as you get to the full amount. Take as much time as you need. The most common side effects of too many supplements will be headache, nausea, and diarrhea. If this should happen to you, simply decrease the number of supplements you are taking and go more slowly. Rarely someone may be allergic to a particular supplement. Should that be the case for you, switch to one I recommend in the second tier. To maintain proper blood levels, supplements need to be taken several times throughout the day, at regular intervals. Nutritional supplements are not like medications that are specially formulated to be time-released. Do not forget a dose and then double up at the next meal. That won't do you any good and you will be wasting money. If you forget a dose, wait until the next regular dose time.

In addition, if I recommend that you take something on an empty stomach, and you forget this aspect, take the supplement anyway. Certain supplements are absorbed better without food in your stomach; they will still be absorbed with food, just not as effectively, so take them.

The treatment I employ for allergies and other similar disorders is close to my program for asthma. I believe that many of these conditions are based on the same underlying problem—an overgrowth of candida, causing a weakening of the immune system. Also, your body undergoes many of the same responses to allergens. Asthma just manifests itself with breathing difficulties and lung damage over time, whereas allergies manifest in a variety of ways you are all too familiar with. The inflammatory response mechanism is the same, and therefore many of the same treatments can be utilized. I am not suggesting that these are the same diseases, but the underlying cause is the same in my opinion.

Once those problems are addressed, you are bound to have fewer allergy-type symptoms. The conditions I have treated with these very similar programs include allergic rhinitis, sinusitis, hives, eczema, psoriasis, and even acne. Therefore, if you have any of those problems and do not have asthma, please read this chapter and follow the nutritional supplement guidelines outlined here.

Since an overgrowth of candida is the main problem in anyone suffering from allergies or the skin conditions that I mentioned, the first place to start is with a proper diet. Please follow the healing-phase dietary guidelines for either losing weight (chapter 9), if need be, or the regular healing-phase diet (chapter 8) if you don't need or have no desire to lose weight.

You then need to follow the nutritional supplement guidelines to help combat an overgrowth of candida. I have suggested two tiers of these supplements. The first tier consists of the ones I use most commonly. I only resort to the second tier when I have not seen the results I wish in my patients. Therefore I recommend that you only resort to the second tier if you are either allergic to one of the first-tier supplements or can't tolerate one or more of them for any reason; simply choose one from the second tier as a replacement. These need to be strictly adhered to for the entire three months of the healing phase and through your transition to the breathing-better phase diet.

Once you have completed this course, you can slowly start to reduce the amount, but not the number of supplements you take, by a third. If all is going well, in six months simply reduce the amount, but not the number of supplements, again by a third. The maintenance dose of these supplements should be that final amount. If you find that your symptoms are getting worse, increase the amount of supplements you are taking and stay with those doses. Another helpful hint I give to my patients is to increase the amount of supplements to full strength a month prior to when you are more susceptible to allergies. Once the season passes, reduce the amount of supplements to their maintenance levels.

Anticandida Supplement Program

Diet is the proper place to start. There aren't enough supplements to help cure your yeast overgrowth without addressing your diet first.

You now know what to do, so please follow the diet while implementing this supplement regimen. If you don't follow the diet and take only these supplements, you are not doing the program correctly.

I usually start the program with just the diet and nutritional supplements. Since candida is so difficult to eradicate, sometimes heavier artillery needs to be employed in the form of prescriptive medications. I usually add these only when the yeast symptoms haven't improved and the patient has been compliant for three months. Other practitioners may add antifungal medications much earlier in the process. They do carry an inherent risk as do any medications, so I try to use them as a last resort. If you are still experiencing symptoms and have been compliant with your diet and nutritional supplement program for three months, I will explain the drugs I use and perhaps you will be able to convince your doctor to prescribe them for you, should you need them.

Top-Tier Anticandida Supplements

Probiotics

These are the opposite of antibiotics—probiotics are beneficial bacteria that live in our gut and are commonly destroyed by the antibiotics we take regularly—by prescription, or through the residue of antibiotics the animals we eat are fed. The imbalance in our gut also can be brought about through the chlorine and fluoride in the tap water we consume. Bad diet and stress contribute to this imbalance as well. Therefore, it is essential to replenish our gut with good bacteria.

There are many different kinds of good bacteria, but I use three most often in my patients. They are lactobacillus acidophilus, bifidobacterium, and lactobacillus bulgaricus. One I use less frequently is laterospora.

Lactobacillus acidophilus: Most people call this acidophilus. It is the most common one found in many nutritional supplements used for this purpose and is most commonly in the small intestine and the vagina. This bacterium helps in immune stimulation by helping the body make interferon, and it also inhibits the growth of candida, *E. coli,* and other harmful bacteria.

Bifidobacterium: This is the most abundant beneficial bacterium in our bodies. Found primarily in the large intestine, it helps lower cholesterol, prevent food poisoning, digest lactose, lower blood levels of ammonia, and aid in the production of many B vitamins.

Bulgaricus: This also may help to stimulate the immune system.

Laterospora: This has been shown to be especially helpful against candida.

Many probiotic preparations contain fructooligosaccharide (FOS), a sugar that generally is not absorbed by the body and that helps beneficial bacteria grow more quickly and efficiently. FOS is in onions, barley, asparagus, and garlic, but you cannot get enough FOS in those foods if you need a therapeutic dosage. A supplement containing FOS may be helpful.

Recommended dosage: Make sure that the supplement you use contains at least the first three strains I discussed, and that what it has in it has been shown to be beneficial in humans. Try to avoid milk-based varieties; many people are sensitive to those strains. Take your supplement before every meal, in a capsule that has at least 1 billion live, active units. The one I use in my practice, "Dr. Ohira's 12 Plus," contains TH10, a potent strain of beneficial bacteria and eleven other hardy strains, along with FOS in a completely vegetarian capsule. Research has been done on this product and that is why I recommend it.

Grapefruit Seed Extract

One of the flavonoids in grapefruit, this helps break down the candida cell wall. I use this in every patient in the dose of 200 to 400 mg three times each day with meals. Its brand name is Paramycocidin or PCN-200. It is very beneficial, and I consider it my first line of therapy.

Caprylic Acid

This is a naturally occurring, medium-chain fatty acid used to fight microorganism, and especially fungal, overgrowth. It is naturally produced in the body in small amounts, and is also in butter, coconut oil, and palm oil. I use this in the dose of 100 mg three times per day with each meal.

Garlic

Garlic has been known to have medicinal properties for as long as recorded time. Garlic contains amino acids, various vitamins and trace minerals, flavonoids, enzymes, and at least two hundred additional compounds. One of them is sulfur-based and is believed to be the antifungal component. Allicin is not the active ingredient for our purposes, so the allicin content of the product you buy is unimportant. I recommend 240 mg three times per day with meals. If that proves to be too much for you because of the garlicky aftertaste, then decrease this amount and slowly build up to it over several weeks.

Those are the four top-tier supplements that I recommend to my patients for yeast or candida. The following are others that I would like to mention that you should only take if you feel you are not getting better fast enough, are allergic to one of these, or want to take more supplements.

Second-Tier Anticandida Supplements

Olive Leaf Extract

This is used to fight most bacterial and viral infections but also plays a role in yeast problems. The active ingredient is oleuropein, which interferes with the production of amino acids essential to the bacteria and fungi. It is also considered to be a strong antioxidant. The dose I recommend is 500 mg three times per day with each meal.

Goldenseal

This herb was first used by Native Americans to fight infections for many years before Western medicine discovered its healing properties. Its active ingredients include alkaloids, berberine, hydrastine, and candidine. It also works well in the sinuses and increases the effectiveness of your body's immune system. Do not use this or any other berberine-containing supplements for extended periods, as they may actually depress immune function when used continuously for extended periods. Use this for less than two weeks at a time. The dose range I recommend is 250 mg three times per day with meals.

Anticandida Supplements for the Cure—Top Tier

1. Probiotics (with or without FOS)—take one that contains beneficial strains for humans before each meal with an approximate dose of 1 billion live cells per capsule. (My recommendation is Ohira's 12 Plus. The dose is one capsule twice per day on an empty stomach.)
2. Grapefruit seed extract—200 to 400 mg three times per day with each meal.
3. Caprylic acid—100 mg three times per day with each meal.
4. Garlic—240 mg three times per day with meals.

Anticandida Supplements for the Cure—Second Tier

1. Olive leaf extract—500 mg three times per day with meals.
2. Goldenseal—250 mg three times per day with meals. Use this for less than two weeks at a time.

Anticandida Medications

If you haven't improved with the recommended nutritional supplements—either symptoms have not gone away, or you can't digest them—you may want to ask your physician for some of the following medications. They can be very beneficial, but many have side effects, so I use them only as a last resort. Give the cure three months to work. You should be following the diet and taking the supplements recommended for candida and those recommended for your particular condition. If you have done this and still are not where you want to be symptomatically, only then would I suggest you try one of these drugs, under the advice of your physician.

There are five drugs currently on the market that I recommend be used to treat candida. They are nystatin, Nizoral (ketoconazole), Diflucan (fluconazole), Sporonox (itraconazole), and Lamisil (terbinafine). Another, amphotericin B, is too toxic to be discussed.

Although these drugs have side effects, if used correctly they can be safe and effective in helping to wipe out your yeast problem.

Nystatin

This was first discovered in the 1940s, and I consider it to be the safest of all the drugs used to treat candida. It is not readily absorbed in the bloodstream, and when taken in recommended doses is passed unchanged in the stool, which means it works in the precise spot needed without affecting anything else systemically. It is considered virtually nontoxic and is even recommended for infants and pregnant women. I usually recommend this in a dose of 500,000 to 1 million units three times per day. Because of some adverse "die-off" reactions that may occur, I usually start the patient with 500,000 units per day and increase the dose gradually over the course of two weeks until they are up to the recommended dose. This is also available in powder, which can be difficult to take, and in an oral suspension loaded with sugar, which can defeat the whole purpose. Stick to the capsules.

The next four drugs work by preventing the yeast cells from growing and inhibit the transformation of the spore forms of yeast to the mycelial form. These mycelia can grow into your gut, causing it to become leaky.

Nizoral (Ketoconazole)

This was first introduced in 1981. I use this drug rarely because I have found others to be tolerated better. Side effects of this medication include elevated liver enzymes; therefore, liver function tests (simple blood tests) should be performed before starting this and periodically throughout treatment. The usual dose is 200 mg per day for one month.

Diflucan (Fluconazole)

This was first used in the United States in 1990 and was used in Europe for many years before that. I have found this to be very safe in my patients and is the drug I use most commonly to treat yeast in patients who do not respond to Nystatin. Side effects can include headache, digestive upsets, and abnormalities in liver function. I almost always take a baseline reading of these just to be safe, but have never found them to elevate, even in patients who took this for weeks or months. I use this drug in the dose of 100 mg per day for about a month. Although I have never seen any side effects, I will not use it for more than a month's duration at a time. I may resume it after a two-week interval, however, if symptoms have not completely resolved.

Sporonox (Itraconazole)

This was released in 1993. It has a broader range of function, meaning that it treats many more kinds of yeast than Diflucan, but since both are effective in candida, I almost always use Diflucan instead of this medication. The most common side effects are gastrointestinal upset and headaches as well as abnormal liver function.

Lamisil (Terbinafine)

I have never used this medication to treat candida. Its mechanism of action is similar to the drugs described and so is likely to be as effective as any of the others. It is given in a dose of 250 mg per day for four weeks.

These drugs appear to be safe and well tolerated if used in small doses and monitored frequently. Please ask your physician to prescribe one for you if you are not able to get relief in ways I have described as first lines of therapy. It is entirely possible that you will need one of these medications if your yeast infection is of a long-standing or particularly severe type. Most allergy or asthma sufferers will have a moderate-to-severe case of yeast, and one of these medications may be necessary if you aren't completely better by the end of the cure.

Allergy Supplement Program

Top-Tier Allergy Supplements

Many nutrients address the symptoms of allergies: runny nose; stuffy nose; and watery, itchy eyes. I am going to describe the ones I most commonly use and their dosage schedule, followed by others you may want to try if your symptom relief is not adequate or if there are some that you cannot tolerate. I will divide them into top and second tiers. The top-tier allergy supplements I recommend are:

Alphabetic

This is a multiple vitamin and a brand name. I have found it to be a superior multivitamin because it is formulated to create optimum antioxidant protection. It contains many minerals and antioxidant vitamins in a once-a-day form that I find refreshing for my patients. The goal is to increase the effectiveness of the immune system and to decrease inflammation. A good antioxidant program can do that, and I have found this multivitamin to be the best of its kind in that regard.

Vitamin C

This vitamin is a cornerstone of our health and is one of the basics. Humans are one of the few species on the planet who cannot synthesize their own vitamin C. If you follow the animal models, most animals make 30 mg per kilogram of body weight per day. If the average human is 150 pounds or 70 kg, we should take about 2,000 mg per day. When under stress, these same animals produce up to seven times that amount, and since allergies and asthma cause chronic stress, it might even be necessary for us to be taking more than what I recommend. I recommend to my patients that they take at least 1,000 mg three times per day with meals.

Vitamin A

This is also a mainstay of therapy. Vitamin A is used for healthy reproduction, blood sugar balance, and defense mechanisms. It is one of the best anti-inflammatory nutrients because of its ability to help the immune system. Its importance for the person with allergies or asthma is that it works particularly well in the mucous membranes of the gastrointestinal tract, helping to heal the problems caused by an overgrowth of yeast organisms. Because of its ability to work on mucous membranes, this vitamin can aid in sinus and other respiratory infections. I recommend 10,000 IU three times per day with meals for three months. Take one month off, then resume and continue to alternate dosage in this way throughout the breathing-better phase of the cure.

Vitamin B_{12}

This can be manufactured in the body by the beneficial bacteria in the gut. Most allergy sufferers have an imbalance in this area, and it is important to add this to the regimen. There is research to document its effectiveness in helping to stop the inflammatory response. I recommend 1,000 mcg per day in the morning on an empty stomach.

Pantethine

This is a member of the B-complex family of vitamins. Many patients get this confused with pantothenic acid. The two are basically the same, because once you take in pantothenic acid it is converted to pantethine, which is then converted to coenzyme A—a very important substance. While you can take pantothenic acid, I recommend that you take pantethine, since it has been shown to produce twice as much coenzyme A in the body as pantothenic acid. Coenzyme A is the basis for the production of hemoglobin, bile, adrenal steroids, and cholesterol. Because of its relationship to the formation of adrenal steroids and because steroid drugs are used for the treatment of allergies, I highly recommend this as part of your nutrient regimen. I recommend 300 mg three times per day with meals for allergy sufferers.

Quercetin

This bioflavonoid is very closely related to vitamin C and is in the rind of most citrus fruits. Since most of us don't eat the rind, we must take this in supplement form. Quercetin is one of nature's best antihistamines. It also has anti-inflammatory properties by fighting off the enzyme that neutralizes cortisone, a natural steroid. I recommend 1,000 mg three times per day with meals.

Magnesium

More than three hundred different enzymes in our bodies depend on this very important mineral, yet the majority of us are deficient in it. That is usually the fault of our diets since it is not in any of the foods commonly associated with the standard American diet. Magnesium helps our body to rid itself of the toxins we consume and face daily; also, as we get older, we tend to absorb fewer nutrients.

Preparations of magnesium include orotate, citrate, oxide, and tau-rate. I use orotate or taurate; I feel they are more absorbable and may create higher blood levels. I recommend 500 mg three times per day with meals. Also, they are less likely to induce diarrhea, a possible side effect of magnesium.

AHCC (Active Hexose Correlated Compound)

This is one of the newest supplements available to the U.S. market. It has been used since 1983 in Japan, where its primary use is in cancer treatment. It greatly reduces side effects of chemotherapy and signifi-cantly increases the quality of life and the life expectancy of those with cancer. It is used in more than seven hundred hospitals in Japan, where it has been extensively studied.

AHCC works by significantly helping the immune system do its job—critical for anyone with allergy or asthma. This supplement has not been shown to overstimulate the immune system, so it can be taken every day. I recommend 500 mg once per day with meals.

Second-Tier Allergy Supplements

Resort to these supplements only if you are allergic to any of the top-tier ones, or if you are not getting the relief you need.

Fish Oils

These are good fats I have discussed and are also known as omega-3 fatty acids. They can suppress inflammation. It is important that the ratio of omega-3s to omega-6 fatty acids be kept in a 1:1 ratio in our bodies. Because most of us consume too many omega-6 fatty acids in our diets, eicosanoids, chemicals in our body, are produced, which can lead to an increased inflammatory response. Our goal in curing your allergies is to decrease inflammation any way we can, and taking in omega-3s is one of the best ways to do this.

The essential fatty acids supplement you take should contain high levels of EPA (eicosapentaenoic acid) and DHA (docosahexaenoic acid). Look for a supplement that contains these two in either a 2:1 or a 3:1 ratio. The usual dose is 500 mg per pill. Some people find that these give them a fishy aftertaste; some preparations add a fruit-flavored extract to help disguise the taste. Fish oils are also helpful in the prevention and treatment of heart disease. I recommend 1,000 mg three times per day with meals.

Vitamin E

This has been shown to be effective in a variety of different disease states and is one of the best antioxidants we know of. In several studies, the lung function of patients improved in proportion to the amount of vitamin E they consumed. I recommend 400 IU twice per day as all others with meals.

Selenium

This is another powerful antioxidant. It is a trace mineral lacking in most of our diets. One of the few ways to get selenium is by taking it in pill form. It has also been shown to work as an anti-inflammatory agent and this is why I suggest it here. I recommend 50 mcg twice per day as earlier with meals.

Allergy Supplements for the Cure—Top Tier

1. Vitamin C—1,000 mg three times per day with meals.
2. Vitamin A—10,000 IU three times per day with meals.
3. Vitamin B$_{12}$—1,000 mcg per day with meals.
4. Pantethine—300 mg three times per day with meals.
5. Quercetin—1,000 mg three times per day with meals.
6. Magnesium—500 mg three times per day with meals.
7. AHCC—500 mg once per day with meals.
8. Alphabetic—1 tablet per day in the mornings.

Allergy Supplements for the Cure—Second Tier

1. Fish oils—1,000 mg three times per day with meals.
2. Vitamin E—400 IU twice per day with meals.
3. Selenium—50 mcg twice per day with meals.

Skin Condition Supplement Program

Top-Tier Skin Condition Supplements

In my experience, the program outlined in this book is very effective for those who suffer with any of the most common skin conditions, such as eczema, hives, psoriasis, and acne. However, there are a few additional nutritional supplements that I recommend specifically for those conditions. If you are reading this book for skin issues, then follow the recommended healing-phase diet program, add the anticandida supplements, add the allergy top-tier supplements, and then add the top-tier skin condition supplements I recommend here. If you are allergic to any of these, or just feel you need more, then refer to the second tier.

Vitamin A

I recommend this in a dose of 20,000 IU three times per day with meals. Take this high dosage for the three-month healing phase, stop for a month, and then continue in this alternating pattern.

Vitamin D_3

This is recommended in a dose of 800 IU three times per day with meals. This has been shown to be very helpful in skin disorders. Again, stop this after three months, take one month off, and then resume in this alternating pattern.

Zinc

This is an important component of every cell in our body. It also plays a critical role in the functioning of our immune systems. Studies have shown that if you build up your zinc stores, your skin will improve. I recommend 30 mg three times a day with meals.

Copper

To keep the proper balance of zinc and copper in your body, take 1 mg three times a day with meals if you follow the dosage recommendation for zinc.

Fish Oils

I recommend 1,000 mg three times per day with meals.

Pantothenic Acid

Although this has been upstaged by pantethine, it is important in itself for skin problems. Since this is a B vitamin, a high dose is quite safe and I recommend up to 1,500 mg three times per day with meals. If you have acne, you may want to increase this dose to 2,000 mg three times per day with meals.

Second-Tier Skin Condition Supplements

Beta-Carotene

This functions as an antioxidant. Since this is in the carotenoid family, it has similar effects in the body as the B-complex family of nutrients and can be effective against inflammation. I recommend 25,000 IU per day with meals.

Manganese

This trace mineral works on a variety of functions in the body, including having an anti-inflammatory response. I recommend a dose range of 15 mg three times per day with each meal.

Skin Condition Supplements for the Cure—Top Tier

1. Vitamin A—20,000 IU three times per day with meals.
2. Vitamin D_3—800 IU three times per day with meals.
3. Zinc—30 mg three times per day with meals.
4. Copper—1 mg three times per day with meals.
5. Fish oils—1,000 mg three times per day with meals.
6. Pantothenic acid—1,500 to 2,000 mg three times per day with meals.

Skin Condition Supplements for the Cure— Second Tier

1. Beta-carotene—25,000 IU per day with meals.
2. Manganese—15 mg three times per day with meals.

Many other nutrients play a role in the treatment of allergies and common skin conditions; I have noted those I use daily in my practice. Chinese herbs, homeopathy, and acupuncture also have been shown to help.

The Allergy and Asthma
Cure Step Seven: Review

1. If you are reading this book for allergies, rhinitis, sinusitis, or other skin conditions, your first step is to follow the healing-phase diet.
2. Keep your symptom questionnaire.
3. Start the anticandida supplement regimen.
4. Start the allergy supplement regimen.
5. If you have any skin disorder such as hives, psoriasis, eczema, or acne, add the skin condition supplements to your regimen.
6. If you have any skin disorder, also include the top-tier allergy supplements.

12

Nutritional Supplements to Treat Asthma: The Allergy and Asthma Cure Step Eight

Nutritional supplements are just as important to the asthma portion of the cure as to the allergies. As previously mentioned, two issues must be addressed in treating allergies or asthma, including sinusitis, eczema, hives, and other very common inflammatory conditions. The first involves candida—the underlying common problem associated with all of these conditions. The second issue is individualized to specific problems. Therefore, anyone reading this book needs to heed the anticandida recommendations, and then follow the recommendations for specific allergy or asthma problems.

Asthma Supplement Program

Many nutritional supplements and other treatments have been used to treat these conditions. I am going to present you with the program I use as well as give you information on other approaches should you not be as successful as you would like using my program.

I recommend that you take the supplements as suggested for the entire healing phase of the diet and through your transition to the breathing-better phase. Then simply reduce the amount of supplements by a third once you have completed the two phases. After an additional six months, reduce the amount of supplements by another third—that will be your maintenance dose of supplements. If you are prone to allergies or asthma at a particular time of year, increase your dose of supplements to their original level one month prior to exposure, then decrease them to maintenance level after that time has passed.

Since many of the supplements will be similar to the ones I described in chapter 11, I will not repeat the description of the supplement unless something is significantly different.

First start with the anticandida supplements. As detailed in chapter 11:

Top-Tier Anticandida Supplements

1. Probiotics (with or without FOS): Take a supplement that contains beneficial strains for humans before each meal with an approximate dose of 1 billion live active units per capsule. (My recommendation is Ohira's 12 Plus in a dose of one capsule twice per day.)
2. Grapefruit seed extract: 200 to 400 mg three times per day with each meal.
3. Caprylic acid: 100 mg three times per day with each meal.
4. Garlic: 240 mg three times per day with meals.

Second-Tier Anticandida Supplements

1. Olive leaf extract: 500 mg three times per day with meals.
2. Goldenseal: 250 mg three times per day with meals. Use this for less than two weeks at a time.

Top-Tier Asthma Supplements

Many supplements have been used to treat asthma. I am going to describe the ones I most commonly use and their dosage schedule, followed by others that you may want to try if your relief is not adequate or if you find you can't tolerate a particular supplement.

Vitamin C

For asthma I recommend 1,000 mg three times per day with meals. At this dosage, vitamin C can act as an antihistamine. Several studies have shown that a daily vitamin C dose of 1 to 2 g can improve lung function and decrease the incidence of asthma attacks. The same dose can protect the bronchial passages from cold temperatures, hay fever, and smog. As mentioned earlier, 2 g of vitamin C before exercise can dramatically decrease the incidence of exercise-induced asthma attacks.

Vitamin A

Vitamin A works particularly well in the mucous membranes of the gastrointestinal tract, helping to heal the problems caused by an overgrowth of yeast organisms.

I recommend this in rather high dosage: 20,000 IU three times per day with meals. This is a fat-soluble vitamin, which means that your body will store it. Too much vitamin A can cause liver damage, but if your body is utilizing it to help you heal, or is deficient in it, you need the recommended dosage; take it for three months only. I have never seen any problem with the thousands of patients that I treat in this way. Note that beta-carotene is not effective for this portion of the treatment.

Magnesium

Magnesium is a key ingredient in treating asthma. Even conventional medical journals support the use of intravenous magnesium to treat an acute asthmatic attack. Magnesium has been shown to diminish wheezing by helping the bronchial muscles to relax. It does the same thing for the muscles of our arteries, which is why magnesium is so important in controlling blood pressure. I recommend magnesium at 500 mg three times per day with meals.

Pantethine

Pantethine is important to the adrenal glands, which produce glucocorticoids, one of the mainstays of conventional asthma therapy. Pantethine may be able to stimulate your own body's production of cortisol. Pantethine can then help decrease inflammation and reduce reliance on prescription drugs. Pantethine also can help promote the growth of the beneficial bacteria discussed earlier.

The dose I use is 300 to 450 mg three times per day with meals.

Fish Oils

These are vitally important for anyone with asthma. I recommend 1,500 mg three times per day with each meal.

Quercetin

Since asthma has such a strong allergic component, this must be part of your regimen. I recommend this in the dose of 500 mg three times per day with each meal.

Vitamin D_3

This form of vitamin D functions as a hormone in the body, helps to absorb calcium, and acts as a natural anti-inflammatory agent.

I recommend this in a dose of 400 IU three times per day with meals, for the three months that you are taking the cure. I have used it in thousands of patients at this dose level without any adverse side effects. If you have any questions, please confer with your personal physician.

Pycnogenol

This is a pine bark extract clinically proven to decrease inflammation. Take 100 mg per day.

Calcium AEP (Colamine Phosphate)

This isn't really calcium at all. Therefore, if you are taking calcium, you will still need to take this. This supplement works as a membrane stabilizer and thus is invaluable in asthma patients. (Most problems from the histamine chain reaction are from destabilization of the membranes.) Colamine phosphate is used most commonly, however, in autoimmune disorders such as multiple sclerosis, lupus, and even thyroid disease. Since there may be an autoimmune component to asthma, all the more reason to use colamine phosphate.

This is best used intravenously, but since that is inconvenient for most patients, it can be used in oral form; I recommend 120 mg three times per day with meals.

Calcium

Calcium is the body's most abundantly stored mineral and is vital for everyone. Make certain that you are also taking the correct amount of magnesium and vitamin D to ensure that the calcium is properly absorbed. Calcium intake has long-term benefits, but you must start early to delay bone loss, which may start in females as young as twenty years.

I do not recommend milk as a calcium source because of its high sugar and phosphorus content. Also, a low-carbohydrate diet will not leach calcium out of your bones.

I have found that calcium in the form of citrate or aspartate is absorbed most easily and is best tolerated. You can find these in your local health food store. I recommend 400 mg three times per day with meals.

AHCC (Active Hexose Correlated Compound)

I recommend 500 mg twice per day with meals.

Supplements for Asthma—Top Tier

1. Vitamin C—1,000 mg three times per day with meals.
2. Vitamin A—20,000 IU three times per day with meals.
3. Magnesium (preferable orotate or taurate)—500 mg three times per day with meals.
4. Pantethine (not pantothenic acid)—300 to 450 mg three times per day with meals.
5. Fish oils—1,500 mg three times per day with meals.
6. Quercetin—500 mg three times per day with meals.
7. Vitamin D—400 IU three times per day with meals.
8. Calcium AEP—120 mg three times per day with meals.
9. Calcium—in the form of citrate or aspartate, preferably; take this 400 mg three times per day with meals.
10. Pycnogenol—50 mg twice per day with meals.
11. AHCC—500 mg twice per day with meals.

Second-Tier Asthma Supplements

I have found that most patients never need to go to this level of therapy. However, some second-tier asthma supplements may be appropriate if you are not getting the relief you desire or if you are allergic or sensitive to some of the top-tier asthma supplements. The following supplements are ones I recommend most frequently.

DHEA

This is a very controversial supplement; I feel that it should be taken under the strict guidance of a physician. Its level must be monitored through a blood test. Some practitioners use DHEA in place of prednisone and consider it a natural form of that drug. It is also considered to be an antiaging hormone. Here I want to mention its possible effects on the person with asthma.

DHEA is naturally found in each one of us. Its level can be measured in the blood, and gets lower as we age. It forms all the other sex and steroid hormones in our body, which is why it may be important in asthma—as it may allow the body to produce more of its own steroid hormones, which are anti-inflammatory. If you do take it, please have your levels checked and monitored. It may produce side effects ranging from abnormal hair growth in women to lower HDL ("good") cholesterol levels in men. Most physicians who prescribe DHEA specify a dose range of 50 to 150 mg per day, best taken on an empty stomach.

Pregnenolone

This hormone, from which DHEA is derived, is naturally found in our bodies. It works as an anti-inflammatory agent without metabolic side effects. I use this only for my steroid-dependent asthma patients. If you take pregnenolone, please see a physician who can closely monitor you; blood levels would need to be checked before you start and while you are on this supplement. The recommended dose is 60 mg three times per day, best taken on an empty stomach.

Taurine

This amino acid, naturally produced in the body in small amounts, is used for many medical conditions other than asthma. It works as a natural diuretic. Regular usage of taurine may help the immune system, and it can begin to act as an antioxidant. Because our lungs are so exposed to free radicals, this may play a protective role. Taurine also can help diminish some of the excess fluid that accumulates in our nasal and breathing passages. I recommend this in a dose of 500 mg three times per day, best taken before meals, on an empty stomach.

N-Acetyl Cysteine

This form of the amino acid cysteine helps to raise glutathione levels in the body and works as an antioxidant. It is used in conventional medicine in the form of inhalers to ward off asthma attacks. It may help to break up mucus. I recommend this in the dose of 500 mg three times per day, best taken on an empty stomach.

Licorice Root Extract

This herbal product, with the chemical name glycyrrhizin, has anti-inflammatory properties and may be used as an expectorant. It is also used to slow down the body's breakdown of steroid medications; because of this action, licorice is sometimes implicated in raising blood pressure. If you are taking any steroid, please consult your physician before using this. I recommend 100 mg three times per day with meals, but please consult your physician before taking this supplement.

Grape Seed Extracts

These contain bioflavonoids called proanthocyanidins (PCOs), which neutralize free radicals very effectively. PCOs also have an anti-inflammatory effect; thus it is in my list for asthma. I recommend 25 mg three times per day with meals.

Supplements for Asthma—Second Tier

1. DHEA—take this only under the guidance of a qualified physician in the dose range of 50 to 150 mg per day; best taken on an empty stomach.
2. Pregnenolone—take this only under the guidance of a physician in the dose range of 60 mg three times per day; best taken on an empty stomach.

3. Taurine—500 mg three times per day; best taken on an empty stomach.
4. N-acetyl cysteine—500 mg three times per day; best taken on an empty stomach.
5. Licorice root extract—100 mg three times per day with meals.
6. Grape seed extract—25 mg three times per day with meals.

There are other, nonconventional ways to treat asthma. I do not use these simply because I am not trained in their use and have found my cure to be quite effective in almost all my patients. Some of the other modalities include acupuncture, homeopathy, and NAET (Nambudripad allergy elimination technique).

I want you to follow the diet I have outlined and take the top-tier supplements for candida and for asthma. That really should be all you need to get the amazing benefits my patients have. Although it may seem I am asking you to do a lot when all conventional medicine asks you to do is puff a few times per day and take a few pills, I wouldn't have written this book if it weren't for all the patients who have turned to me, unhappy with how they were feeling. They inspired me to create a program that works and to share it with all of you. I hope my program works as well for you as it does for my patients. Good luck!

The Allergy and Asthma Cure
Step Eight: Review

1. Follow the healing-phase diet.
2. Begin taking the anticandida supplements.
3. Add supplement recommendations to your program as appropriate—allergies, asthma, eczema, etc.
4. Keep your symptom questionnaire to help you determine which food/supplements are appropriate for you.
5. Gradually build up the number of supplements you take for best effectiveness; it may take several weeks to be on the full number of supplements I recommend.
6. If your symptoms do not completely resolve by the end of the three-month period, or if you can't take the antiyeast supplements, discuss with your doctor the possibility of taking one of the antifungal medications.

7. If you need to take one of the medications, follow the rest of the suggested parts of the cure until the course of medication has been completed.

8. Supplement dosages I suggest are appropriate for most people. Children should take less, and adults heavier than 300 pounds should increase by one extra dose per day.

9. If you forget to take something that is appropriate on an empty stomach, take it anyway, as it will still be absorbed, although not as effectively.

10. Continue with the supplement program as recommended for the three months of the healing phase and then throughout your entire transition to the breathing-better phase. At that point, if all is well, reduce the amount, not the number, of different supplements by a third. In another six months, reduce the amount of supplements by another third, which will be your maintenance dose of supplements.

11. During times of the year when you may be particularly prone to allergy or asthma attacks, increase the amount of supplements you take to their original dose one month prior to your season. Reduce to the maintenance level once your season has passed.

12. If there is a supplement that I suggest you keep close tabs on, please follow only the recommended dosage.

13. Use these suggestions along with the advice of your regular doctor.

14. Feel better.

PART IV

The Allergy and Asthma Cure Meal Plans and Recipes

13

Meal Plans

I am including meal plans in this book because I have asked you to undertake a drastic change in your diet. These meal plans, and the recipes in chapter 14, include foods that are delicious. Before you start the program, eliminate everything from your house or apartment that you cannot eat. This will make it far easier for you to stay with the cure. You immediately eliminate any source of cheats or temptations from at least one area of your life. Review the diet program that you are going to follow and then plan a shopping day. Take your time, walk through the store, read labels. The foods are going to be different, but it is only a matter of time before you become accustomed to this new way of shopping and to your new diet.

In addition, if you work, think about where you eat lunch and if you snack. Find appropriate places to eat or buy foods that allow you to stay with your program. If this is impossible, then carefully plan alternatives, such as bringing food from home. The people who do the best on this program are those who spend some time getting organized and then do it correctly. This program may take some advance preparation, so don't set yourself up to fail. Set yourself up to succeed by taking the time to set the foundation before you embark on the cure. Don't try to do this without preparing for it, especially in the first two weeks. You can do this; many have before you and are breathing easier because of it.

The menus in this chapter were created for the strictest person on the program. Therefore, anyone reading this book should be able to enjoy the items on these menus. The recipes may be somewhat unique, but I wanted to give you ideas for when you need something special. These will also serve as jumping-off points for your own ideas. I did this because I assume (maybe wrongly!) that you already know how to steam vegetables, bake a plain piece of fish, grill a steak, or pour a bowl of yeast-free cereal. I wanted these menus to be more exciting. I wanted you to see that eating in this manner need not be boring or bland. All of the recipes for the dishes I mention here are in chapter 14, except those marked with an asterisk and those for the second week. I have even included appetizers, soups, and a few more breakfast and dinner entrées to help whet your appetite for the program. For dessert I recommend diet Jell-O, $1/2$ protein bar or shake, or even better, just get into the habit of not having dessert. For yeast-free dessert recipes please refer to the many cookbooks on yeast-free foods currently available.

Happy eating and good luck!

Week 1; Day 1

Breakfast: Vegetable Timbale
Lunch: Seafood Salad
Dinner: Chicken Medallions with Spring Sauce
Side: Green Rice
Vegetable: steamed broccoli with butter*

Day 2

Breakfast: Sausage and Onions
Lunch: Grilled Marinated Chicken on a Bean Bed

---

* There are no recipes in chapter 14 for items marked with an asterisk in this chapter.

Dinner: Shrimp Kabobs with Salsa

Side: Red Pepper Custards

Vegetable: romaine lettuce salad with macadamia nut oil, white wine vinegar, and Italian spices*

DAY 3

Breakfast: Scrambled Eggs with Garlic and Peppers

Lunch: Cold Poached Salmon on a bed of lettuce

Dinner: Lemon Steak

Side: Potato Salad

Vegetable: sautéed Brussels sprouts with pine nuts and marjoram*

DAY 4

Breakfast: Breakfast Lentils and Eggs

Lunch: Nutty Chicken Salad

Dinner: Blind Finches

Side: Stuffed Crooknecks

DAY 5

Breakfast: Salmon Hash

Lunch: Hamburger with Pizzazz

Dinner: Savory Chicken Breasts

Side: Tasty Cauliflower

Side: quinoa with macadamia nut oil dressing*

DAY 6

Breakfast: Middle Eastern Herb Omelette

Lunch: Salad Plate

Dinner:Lemon-Scented Shrimp

Side: Spaghetti

Vegetable: sautéed cucumbers and zucchini with lemon and olive oil dressing*

DAY 7

Breakfast: Popeye's Delight

Lunch: Eastern Beef Salad

Dinner: Zesty Pork Loins

Side: sweet potato cakes

Vegetable: spinach salad with macadamia nut oil and crumbled pepper goat cheese (if permitted) dressing*

WEEK 2; DAY 1

Breakfast: 2 scrambled eggs with 1 Ry-vita (or similar) whole-grain cracker

Lunch: chicken salad over a bed of greens

Dinner: grilled rib eye steak

Side: $1/_2$ cup of brown rice with macadamia nut oil drizzled over it

Vegetable: salad with olive oil, pine nuts, and 2 diced olives

DAY 2

Breakfast: spelt cereal with 1 tablespoon of cream and 4 ounces of water, with 1 ounce of chopped pecans sprinkled on top

Lunch: grilled tuna over a bed of lettuce

Dinner: barbecued hamburger (no bun)

Side: walnut and millet salad

Vegetable: sautéed broccoli and cauliflower heated in macadamia nut oil

DAY 3

Breakfast: asparagus/bacon and egg salad

Lunch: sliced turkey rolled around shredded peppers

Dinner: grilled pork chops

Side: buckwheat with almonds

Vegetable: frisé salad with endive and macadamia nut oil dressing with fines herbes

DAY 4

Breakfast: salmon salad on yeast-free whole-grain bread

Lunch: tuna salad on a bed of lettuce

Dinner: grilled swordfish

Side: sautéed spinach with whole garlic cloves

DAY 5

Breakfast: unsweetened nut butter on whole-grain cracker with spiced cream cheese

Lunch: grilled chicken breast over a bed of lettuce

Dinner: beef stir-fry with vegetables

Side: salad with macadamia nut oil, cayenne pepper, and stevia dressing

DAY 6

Breakfast: protein shake with 1 tablespoon of unsweetened peanut butter blended together in a blender

Lunch: hamburger with side salad

Dinner: roasted leg of lamb

Side: sautéed green beans with butter and garlic

Vegetables: salad with olive oil and Cajun spices dressing

DAY 7

Breakfast: soy flour pancakes

Lunch: toasted walnut and arugula salad with olive oil, avocado, and sesame seed dressing

Dinner: grilled monkfish

Side: steamed vegetable medley with red pepper flakes

Vegetable: romaine salad with macadamia nut oil, marjoram, thyme, and crushed black peppercorn dressing

Once you start to see how delicious these foods can be, you are going to get the hang of the diet portion of this program quite quickly.

This is a critical part of the cure, and you won't succeed unless you get the diet part correct. Use these meal plans as a place to start—and have an adventure along the way.

14

Recipes

The recipes in this chapter indicate everything you need to prepare each of the first week menu items mentioned in chapter 13, except those marked with an asterisk. There are even extra-tasty recipes for you to serve at dinner parties. Many of these can be made ahead of time and heated when you need them.

BREAKFAST

Breakfast Lentils and Eggs

SERVES 4

$^3/_4$ cup French green lentils
$^1/_2$ lb bacon, sliced into $^1/_4$-inch cubes
1 cup leeks, chopped (use the pale green and white parts only)
1 tbs macadamia nut oil
1 tbs tarragon, minced

2 tbs lemon juice
1 cup celery, chopped
$^1/_2$ tsp olive oil
$^1/_2$ tsp minced garlic
1 10-oz box frozen spinach
8 eggs
salt and pepper to taste

Simmer the lentils in a stockpot, covered by 2 inches of water, until tender, about 20 minutes. Crisp-cook the bacon in a large nonstick skillet. Reserve the drippings in the skillet and remove the bacon to paper towels and drain. Add the leeks and celery to the drippings, and sauté until tender. Remove the skillet from the heat and stir in the lemon juice. Drain the lentils and add them to this vegetable mixture. Season with the minced tarragon, salt, and pepper. Fold in $1/2$ of the cooked bacon bits. Set aside and keep warm.

Sauté the garlic in $1/2$ tsp of olive oil. Add the spinach. Stir the spinach in the oil until thawed and then cover the pan.

Warm 1 tbs of macadamia nut oil in a nonstick skillet. Break 2 eggs in opposite sides of the skillet. Cover and cook until the yolks are runny and the whites are set.

Divide the lentil mixture among 4 plates. Top with spinach and then 2 eggs. Sprinkle with the remaining bacon bits and a grind of fresh black pepper.

* * *

Salmon Hash

SERVES 4

4 large eggs	$1/2$ cup red pepper
4 tbs butter	2 tsp thyme
$1^1/_2$ lb yams	2 sprigs fresh sage
2 bunches scallions	$1/2$ lb boneless, skinless salmon fillet

Bring a skillet of salted water to a gentle simmer. Slip in the salmon fillet and cover the saucepan. Turn off the heat and allow the salmon to cool until you are able to handle the fillet. It should be about half cooked and very rare in the middle. Flake the cooked fish into large chunks and set aside.

Cut the yams into $1/2$-inch-square cubes. Place the cubes in a steamer basket over boiling water. Steam these for 15 minutes or until al dente. Melt the butter in a large skillet, on medium high. Add the yams, chopped scallions, red pepper, and thyme to the skillet. Allow the mixture to brown without disturbing it. Distribute the salmon and minced sage leaves over the potato mixture and flip it to brown the other side. Remove from heat after about 2 minutes. Do not overcook.

While the potato mixture is browning, poach the eggs until the yolk is runny and the white is firm. Divide the salmon and potato mixture among 4 plates and top with a poached egg. Sprinkle with freshly ground pepper and a parsley sprig.

* * *

Middle Eastern Herb Omelette

SERVES 4 TO 6

4 cups loosely packed spinach
1 bunch scallions
$^1/_2$ bunch flat leaf parsley
$^1/_2$ bunch cilantro
1 tbs fresh dill (fronds only)

1 tbs fresh tarragon
1 clove garlic
1 tbs brown rice flour
8 large eggs
$^1/_4$ cup butter, melted

Place the first 7 ingredients into a food processor or blender and whirl until finely chopped. Sprinkle the flour over the minced herbs and pulse twice to combine.

In a separate bowl, beat the eggs until frothy. Add to the herbs mixture and pulse several times to combine. Swirl the butter in a 2-quart casserole dish and then pour in the egg/herb mixture.

Bake in a 350°F oven for 40 to 50 minutes or until the eggs have set to your liking.

* * *

Popeye's Delight

SERVES 4

4 large eggs
1$^1/_2$ lb fresh spinach
4 tbs minced onions
2 tbs butter

$^1/_4$ cup heavy cream
$^1/_8$ tsp nutmeg
pepper to taste

Trim and rinse the spinach. Blanch in boiling, salted water until the leaves just wilt, about 30 seconds. Drain well and blot with a paper towel to remove all moisture.

Melt the butter in a medium saucepan. Add the onions, and sauté until soft and translucent. Add the spinach, cream, and nutmeg, stirring until warmed. Divide the mixture among 4 au gratin dishes. Make a well in the center of each of the mounds of spinach and break one egg into each well. For ease of transfer, place the dishes onto a cookie sheet and put into a 400°F oven for 12 to 15 minutes, depending on your preference for hard or soft yolks. Remove from the oven and sprinkle with freshly cracked pepper.

* * *

Vegetable Timbales

I like to make these ahead of time and use them throughout the week for a quick, tasty breakfast on the run. Also, as a variation, you can mix all of the vegetables for a different flavor.

SERVES 4

$1/_2$ cup cream
1 cup chicken stock
4 eggs
$3/_4$ tsp salt
1 tbs chopped parsley

$1-1^1/_2$ cups well-drained cooked spinach, broccoli, or cauliflower, chopped or put through a food processor

Preheat the oven to 325°F. Combine all the ingredients except the vegetables in a large bowl and beat with a wire whisk. After these ingredients are thoroughly combined, add the vegetables and combine. Pour the mixture into individual ramekins and fill them about $2/_3$ full. Place on a rack in a pan of water and bake in the oven for 20 minutes or longer, depending on the size of your ramekin. They are done when a knife blade inserted into the center of the mold comes out uncoated.

* * *

Scrambled Eggs with Garlic and Peppers

SERVES 2

1 tbs butter
3 eggs
$1/_4$ tsp salt
$1/_8$ tsp pepper

2 tbs cream
1 clove garlic, minced
1 small bell pepper, diced

Melt the butter in a skillet over low heat. Beat all the ingredients except the bell pepper and the garlic in a small bowl until the eggs are uniform in color. Add the garlic and the bell pepper and mix thoroughly. By this time the butter should be melted. Add the mixture to the skillet and slightly increase the heat. As the eggs heat through, shove the eggs around the skillet gently but with accelerating speed, turning them if necessary, until they have thickened.

* * *

Sausage and Onions
SERVES 4

1 tbs olive oil

1$^1/_2$ cups diced onions

8 sausage links (sugar-free)

Heat the oil in a skillet. Add the onions and cook over a low heat about 15 minutes or until golden. Slit the sausage links down the center and fill them with the onions. Fasten with wooden picks. Broil slowly on both sides until done.

❋ ❋ ❋

Fun Sausage and Scramblers
SERVES 6

1 lb pork sausage (spicy and sage if available—these should not contain sugar)

$^1/_2$ cup uncooked oats

$^1/_2$ tsp salt

$^1/_2$ tsp sage (rubbed or powdered type)

$^1/_2$ cup ricotta cheese, twirled in a food processor

9 eggs

1 tsp salt

dash white pepper

$^1/_4$ cup club soda

fresh parsley or dill

Preheat oven to 350°F. Combine the first 5 ingredients completely. Place 6 ramekins or custard cups on a baking sheet. Press the sausage medley into the cups and bake until fully cooked and firm, about 45 minutes.

Beat the eggs, salt, pepper, and club soda until frothy. Warm a large skillet and melt the butter. Add the eggs to the skillet and stir until almost set. Remove from the pan and spoon the eggs into each sausage cup (the eggs will continue to cook even off the heat). Garnish with a sprig of fresh parsley or dill.

❋ ❋ ❋

Nesting Eggs
SERVES 4

$^1/_2$ cup brown rice

1 chicken bouillon cube

$^1/_4$ cup sliced almonds

5 scallions, chopped (white and light green sections only)

$^1/_2$ tsp Italian seasoning

$^1/_2$ cup ricotta cheese

salt and pepper to taste

Bring one cup of water to a boil in a medium saucepan. Add the brown rice and the bouillon cube. Simmer until the rice is tender, about 20 minutes. Remove from the heat and add the scallions, seasoning, and almonds.

Spray 4 ramekins with olive oil and press $1/4$ of the mixture into each dish, pushing the rice up the side of the dish to form a cup. Break 1 egg into each cup, top with $1/4$ of the ricotta and season with salt and freshly ground pepper. Bake at 350°F until the yolks are set to your liking (12 to 18 minutes).

⊙ ⊙ ⊙

Breakfast Veggie Medley

SERVES 6

1 lb zucchini	1 tsp dill
$1/2$ lb yellow squash	1 cup turkey, diced
1 10-oz package frozen spinach	2 oz cream cheese
1 tsp minced garlic	2 tbs cream
6 eggs	macadamia nut oil in a spray bottle
1 cup cottage cheese	

Spray a large nonstick skillet with macadamia nut oil. Add the zucchini, yellow squash, spinach, and garlic. Cook until the spinach has thawed and heated and the squash is tender, about 8 to 10 minutes. Drain in a colander.

Beat together the eggs, cottage cheese, and dill. Stir in the turkey and the vegetables. In a separate small bowl, mix the cream and the cream cheese. Spray a 9x9 pan with macadamia nut oil and pour in the egg mixture. Dollop the cream cheese over the egg mixture. Bake in a 350°F oven for 30 minutes or until a tester in the center of the dish comes out clean.

Allow the medley to rest for 5 minutes and then slice into 6 wedges.

LUNCH

Seafood Salad

SERVES 4 TO 6

1 lb raw medium shrimp, cleaned and butterflied	1 bay leaf
	1 tsp sea salt
1 lb sea scallops, cut into quarters	5 black peppercorns
$1/2$ lb calamari, cleaned and sliced into rings	1 red pepper, diced
	1 small red onion, finely diced

2 garlic cloves, minced

$^1/_2$ cup olive oil

juice of 2 lemons

$^1/_4$ cup parsley, minced

Bring a large stockpot of water to a rolling boil. Add the bay leaf, peppercorns, and sea salt. Toss in the shrimp, and after $^1/_2$ minute, add the scallops and calamari. Cook an additional $2^1/_2$ minutes. Drain and refresh immediately in an ice bath. Discard the bay leaf and peppercorns.

Put the remaining ingredients in a large glass jar and shake vigorously to mix. Pour the dressing over the seafood mixture.

Allow the salad to rest in the refrigerator for at least 2 hours to meld the flavors and chill.

* * *

Grilled Marinated Chicken on a Bean Bed
SERVES 4

4 boneless, skinless chicken breasts

$^1/_4$ cup olive oil, mixed with $^1/_4$ tsp each salt, minced garlic, and oregano, and $^1/_8$ tsp pepper

2 15-oz cans white cannelli beans

1 red onion, very thinly sliced

$^1/_2$ each red and yellow peppers, thinly sliced

1 cup basil leaves, julienned

2 cloves, minced garlic

$^1/_2$ cup olive oil

2 tbs fresh lemon juice

$^1/_2$ cup parsley, finely minced, divided

Marinate the chicken in the olive oil mixture for at least 1 hour. Discard the marinade. With the grill on high heat, cook the chicken until no longer pink inside, about 6 minutes per side. Remove from grill to a platter and cover with plastic wrap. Cool to room temperature.

In a bowl, mix the beans, peppers, onion, basil, garlic, and $^1/_4$ cup parsley. In a separate bowl, whisk together the lemon juice and olive oil; pour this over the bean mixture and toss to coat.

Divide the beans among the serving plates. Slice the chicken breasts on the diagonal and place them on the beans. Sprinkle with the remaining parsley.

* * *

Cold Poached Salmon

SERVES 4

4 salmon fillets, boned

Using a deep skillet, bring 2 quarts of salted water to a rolling boil. Slip the fillets into the water and immediately reduce the heat to a gentle simmer. Cover the skillet and allow the fillets to simmer for 5 minutes. Remove from the heat and check for doneness. (The timing above will cook the fish to medium. If you prefer your fish fully cooked, increase the simmer to 7 minutes and keep the fish covered after you remove the skillet from the heat.) Remove the fish and cool. Remove any skin or gray matter.

Salsa for Salmon

SERVES 4

2 cucumbers, peeled, seeded, and finely diced

1 small jalapeño, seeded and very finely diced

1 red pepper, seeded and finely diced

juice of 1 lime

$1/4$ cup finely diced red onion

1 tsp cumin

$1/4$ cup cilantro, chopped

Mix all ingredients. Refrigerate 2 hours to blend the flavors. Serve over the cold poached salmon.

Hamburger with Pizzazz

SERVES 4

1 small onion, finely minced

1 tbs macadamia nut oil

2 cloves garlic, finely minced

1 tsp black pepper

$1/2$ tsp nutmeg

1 tsp coriander

2 lb lean ground beef

Sauté the onion in macadamia nut oil until translucent, about 5 minutes. Add garlic and spices and cook for another 5 minutes, until the spices are fragrant.

Combine the spice mixture and the ground beef. Form the mixture into 4 patties. Refrigerate for at least 1 hour.

Grill the patties to desired doneness (about 3 minutes per side for medium). Serve with thinly sliced red onion and lettuce.

Nutty Chicken Salad

SERVES 4 TO 6

2 cups chicken, cooked and diced
1 small red onion, minced
$1/_4$ cup pecans, finely chopped
2 stalks celery, diced

2 tbs parsley, minced
$1/_2$ cup mayonnaise
3 tbs chicken broth

Place the first five ingredients into a large mixing bowl. In a separate small bowl, thin the mayonnaise with the chicken broth and then add this mixture to the chicken. Toss to coat. Check for seasoning and add any necessary salt and pepper. Chill the salad to meld the flavors. Serve over a bed of lettuce.

Eastern Beef Salad

SERVES 4

1 pound top sirloin steak
$1^1/_2$ tbs minced fresh garlic
$1/_4$ tsp red pepper flakes
$1/_4$ tsp black pepper

$1/_2$ tsp garlic powder
$1/_4$ tsp coriander
$1/_8$ tsp salt

Place the garlic and spices on a chopping block. With the flat side of a knife, mash the mixture. With the blade gather the mixture and then mash again, forming a paste.

Rub the paste on both sides of the meat and allow it to rest for 1 hour. Grill to desired doneness and then allow to cool. Slice into thin strips.

8 cups spring salad mix
$1/_4$ cup mint, chopped
1 medium cucumber, seeded and
   sliced

1 bunch scallions, sliced
$1/_2$ cup cilantro, chopped

While the steak is cooling, toss all the above ingredients.

4 tbs fresh lime juice
$1/_3$ cup macadamia nut oil

2 tsp chopped red chili
1 tsp sesame seeds

Whisk together the lime juice, macadamia nut oil, and chopped red chili. Toss the greens with this mixture. Mound the salad on 4 plates and top with the sliced steak. Sprinkle with sesame seeds and serve.

Salad Plate

SERVES 2

1 head endive
1 head radicchio

3 cups spring salad mix

Salad Dressing:

$1/_3$ cup olive oil
3 tbs fresh lemon juice

1 tsp Italian seasoning
salt and pepper to taste

Salad Components:

2 hard-boiled eggs
1 cup cottage cheese
1 cup grilled turkey or chicken,
    sliced

1 cup trimmed, blanched, and
    chilled green beans
4 rings sliced from a red pepper
1 tbs capers
4 canned anchovies

Place the olive oil, fresh lemon juice, and seasonings in a small glass jar with a screw top. Close and shake vigorously. Mix the three salad greens and toss with the dressing. Divide between 2 plates. Decoratively arrange the salad components on the salad, ending with 2 anchovies in an X pattern.

DINNER

Shrimp Kabobs with Salsa

SERVES 4

1 lb large shrimp, peeled and
    cleaned
wooden skewers, soaked in water
    for $1/_2$ hour
$1/_4$ cup macadamia nut oil

$1/_4$ cup fresh lime juice
2 cloves garlic, minced
1 tbs hot sauce
salt and pepper to taste

Combine the macadamia nut oil, lime juice, garlic, hot sauce, and salt and pepper. Toss with the shrimp and then refrigerate for 2 to 3 hours.

Heat the grill. Thread the shrimp onto the skewers and grill them until pink and no longer translucent, about 4 minutes per side. Serve with salsa.

● ● ●

Salsa for Shrimp

SERVES 4

1 cup canned black beans, drained
    and rinsed
2 tbs minced red pepper
3 tbs minced red onion
$^1/_4$ cup cucumber, peeled, seeded,
    and cut into 1$^1/_2$-inch dice
1 tbs diced celery
$^1/_2$ tbs fresh basil, chopped

1 tbs finely minced jalapeño
2 tbs macadamia nut oil
2 tbs lemon juice
1 tsp fresh thyme, chopped
$^1/_4$ tsp cumin
$^1/_4$ tsp chili powder
$^1/_8$ tsp salt and pepper
1 clove garlic, minced

Combine all salsa ingredients and allow the flavors to meld in the refrigerator for 1 hour before serving on the side of the kabobs.

❖ ❖ ❖

Chicken Medallions with Spring Sauce

SERVES 4

4 skinless, boneless chicken
    breasts, pounded flat
$^1/_4$ cup brown rice flour
2 tbs unsalted butter
2 tbs macadamia nut oil

1 lb fresh green asparagus,
    trimmed
$^1/_2$ tsp salt
$^1/_8$ tsp nutmeg
minced parsley for garnish

Blanch the asparagus in boiling water for 7 minutes. Drain. Cut off 1 inch of the tips and reserve. Place the remaining asparagus in the bowl of a food processor. Add the cream, salt, and nutmeg, and process until smooth. Transfer the cream mixture to a small saucepan and bring to a simmer. Allow to thicken.

Heat the butter and the oil in a large skillet. Toss the medallions with the flour. Add the chicken to the oil/butter and cook until done. Season with salt and pepper.

Place the medallions on a serving platter. Coat the medallions with the sauce and then top with the asparagus tips and a sprinkle of minced parsley.

❖ ❖ ❖

Lemon Steak

SERVES 4 TO 6

1 1¹/₂-lb sirloin steak or London
  broil
1 tsp grated lemon zest
¹/₂ cup fresh lemon juice
¹/₃ cup olive oil (specialty food
  stores will have lemon-flavored
  olive oil)

2 tbs minced scallions
2 tsp dry mustard
¹/₄ tsp pepper

Tenderize the meat with a meat mallet. Place in a large freezer zip-type plastic bag. Mix all the remaining ingredients and pour over the steak in the bag. Refrigerate overnight. Drain the marinade into a small saucepan, and bring to a boil. Keep warm.

Grill the steak over high heat to desired doneness (about 6 minutes per side for medium rare). Slice against the grain and spoon a small amount of the marinade over the sliced steak. Serve.

❊ ❊ ❊

Blind Finches

SERVES 4

4 ¹/₃-lb thinly pounded sirloin
  steaks
³/₄ lb bulk pork sausage
¹/₂ cup prepared brown rice or
  kasha
2 tbs minced fresh parsley
2 tbs fresh lemon juice

1 tsp pepper
¹/₂ tsp salt
¹/₄ tsp nutmeg
¹/₄ tsp ground sage
4 tbs butter
¹/₂ cup beef bouillon

In a skillet over medium-high heat, cook the pork sausage until crumbly and brown. Transfer to the bowl of a food processor and add the remaining ingredients except the steaks and the butter. Pulse briefly; you want the rice or kasha and the sausage to break up but not purée.

Lay the steaks on a flat surface. Divide the sausage mixture among the steaks. Pack it with your hands so it does not break up. Roll the steaks jelly roll style, tucking in the sides so you have a compact package. Tie each with kitchen string.

Heat the butter in a nonstick frying pan and add the packages. Brown the meat, turning infrequently. Add the bouillon, cover the pan, and simmer for 15 minutes until cooked through. Remove the packages from the pan, remove string, slice, and pour the pan juices over the meat. Serve.

* * *

Lemon-Scented Shrimp

SERVES 4

1 tbs minced fresh thyme (use lemon thyme if available)	1 tbs macadamia nut oil
	1 tsp cayenne
3 tbs fresh lemon juice	1 lb jumbo shrimp

Mix together the thyme, lemon juice, macadamia nut oil, and cayenne in a glass bowl or plastic zip bag. Peel and butterfly the shrimp, rinse, pat dry, and add to the marinade. Refrigerate for at least 1 hour and up to 2 hours.

Remove the shrimp from the marinade. Thread onto metal kebab skewers tail to top, forming a nugget. Grill over high heat, basting with the remaining marinade. Cook until opaque, about 4 minutes per side. Serve.

* * *

Savory Chicken Breasts

SERVES 4

4 tbs butter	4 boneless, skinless chicken breasts
1$^1/_2$ tbs dry mustard	
$^3/_4$ cup finely ground pecans	1 tbs macadamia nut oil

With a flat meat mallet, pound the chicken breasts to $^1/_4$ inch thick.

Melt 3 tbs of butter and whisk in 1 tbs of dry mustard. Put the pecans on a flat dish. Dip each chicken breast in the mustard mixture and then dredge in the ground pecans.

Melt 1 tbs of butter with the macadamia nut oil. When the pan is medium hot, add the chicken breasts. Cook until golden brown, about 3 minutes per side. Remove the chicken breasts and keep warm. Sprinkle the flour over the drippings, stir, and then pour in the cream/bouillon mixture. Bring to a boil and season with pepper as desired. Spoon the sauce over the chicken breasts and serve.

* * *

Zesty Pork Loins

SERVES 4

1 lb pork tenderloins　　　　　　　2 tbs olive oil

Marinade:

2 cloves garlic, finely minced　　　1 tsp fennel seed, crushed in a
1/2 cup olive oil　　　　　　　　　mortar and pestle
2 limes, juice and zest　　　　　　1/8 tsp red pepper flakes
1 tsp ground cumin　　　　　　　　2 tbs dry mustard

Place all marinade ingredients in a zip-type plastic bag and mix. Add the pork loins, close, and refrigerate overnight.

Remove the tenderloins from the bag, reserving the marinade. Heat the 2 tbs olive oil in a large skillet with a heatproof handle. Brown the pork on all sides, about 2 minutes per side. Pour the marinade over the pork and place in a 375°F oven for 15 minutes; the tenderloins should be lightly pink. Remove from the oven and allow the pork to rest for 5 minutes before slicing. Serve.

❀ ❀ ❀

The following two dinner entrées are not included in the menu chapter. The veal scallops may be substituted for any of the dishes mentioned, but the chicken dish is for when you are able to incorporate cheese back into your program.

Veal Scallops

SERVES 4

1 1/2 lb veal scallops, pounded thin　2 tbs butter
1 tsp salt　　　　　　　　　　　　2 tbs heavy cream
1/2 tsp pepper　　　　　　　　　　1 tsp minced tarragon
4 tbs butter　　　　　　　　　　　1 cup cooked, lump crabmeat
juice of one lemon　　　　　　　　8 spears cooked asparagus

Season the veal scallops with salt and pepper. Heat the butter in a skillet and sauté the scallops until lightly browned on each side. Remove and keep warm.

Add the 2 tbs additional butter to the saucepan, scraping up any brown bits. Add the lemon juice, cream, and tarragon. Simmer until thickened.

Divide the scallops among 4 serving plates. Spoon the sauce over the scallops. Place a 1/4-cup scoop of the crabmeat on each portion of veal. Arrange 2 asparagus spears over each portion and finish with freshly cracked pepper.

❀ ❀ ❀

Stuffed Chicken Breasts

SERVES 6

6 bone-in chicken breasts

6 tbs Dijon mustard

1 10-oz package frozen spinach, thawed and pressed dry

$1/_2$ cup ricotta

$1/_2$ cup minced scallions

$1/_2$ tsp poultry seasoning

Mix the spinach, ricotta, scallions, and poultry seasoning. Season with salt and pepper.

Make a pocket in the breasts and divide the spinach mixture among the 6 breasts. Spread the mustard over the top of each breast. Arrange on a baking sheet.

Bake at 350°F for 25 minutes or until cooked through and golden brown.

SIDE DISHES

Green Rice

SERVES 6

1 cup brown rice

2 cups vegetable broth (a vegetable bouillon cube works well here)

1 bay leaf

2 cups jullienned spinach leaves

3 scallions thinly sliced on the diagonal

1 cup Italian parsley, minced

$1/_4$ cup fresh basil, minced

1 tbs fresh tarragon, minced

$1/_8$ tsp nutmeg

Steam the spinach leaves for 1 minute until just wilted. Set aside. Combine the rice, broth, and bay leaf in a saucepan. Bring the rice to a boil and simmer for 35 minutes. When you are ready to serve, mix the rice, spinach, and all remaining ingredients.

❀ ❁ ❀

Red Pepper Custards

SERVES 6

1 cup water

$1/_2$ cup brown rice

1 15-oz jar red peppers

5 eggs

1 cup heavy cream

1 tbs fresh basil, minced

1 tsp dried dill weed

1 small fresh green bell pepper

olive oil in a spray bottle

Bring the water to a boil in a small saucepan. Add the rice, cover, and simmer until the rice is cooked, about 35 minutes.

Drain the peppers in a colander and blot them dry with a paper towel. Purée the red peppers in a food processor. Measure out $2/3$ of a cup. Reserve the remainder for another use.*

In a medium bowl, whisk together the cream and eggs. Mix in the rice, the puréed peppers, basil, and dill. Season with salt and pepper.

Spray 6 custard cups with olive oil. Cut the green pepper in half, remove the seeds, and with the heel of your hand, flatten the pepper. Using a decorative cutter or a knife, cut shapes from the flattened pepper (such as a small star, multiple tiny diamonds, or a flower). Place the shape in the bottom of the custard cup and then ladle the red pepper mixture evenly among the cups. Put the cups in a baking pan and add 1 inch of hot water.

Bake in a 350°F oven for approximately 45 minutes or until the custard is set in the center (you can test with a cake tester). After you have removed the custards from the oven, allow them to rest for 10 minutes. Run a thin spatula between the custard and the cup. Invert onto a serving plate.

❋ ❋ ❋

Potato Salad

SERVES 6 TO 8

1 large onion, diced	1 tsp cinnamon
3 tbs macadamia nut oil	1 tsp paprika
1$1/2$ lbs yams, peeled, and cut into 1-inch dice	1 tbs freshly grated ginger
	1 lemon, divided use
1 pinch cayenne paper	$1/4$ cup cilantro, minced
1 pinch saffron (if available)	2 tbs macadamia nut oil

In a frying pan, sauté the onion in 3 tbs of macadamia nut oil until tender. Add the yams, all the spices, and the juice from the lemon. Pour in enough water to just cover the yams. Simmer gently for 15 minutes; the yams should be al dente. The water should have transformed to a syrupy sauce. If it is still runny, remove the yams and reduce the sauce. Return the yams to the pan

---

* You can sauté a bit of garlic and onion in olive oil. Add the reserved red pepper purée and a sprinkle of cayenne pepper and salt. Simmer for a few minutes and then serve it over a baked spaghetti squash.

and stir in the zest from the lemon, the cilantro, and 2 tbs of macadamia nut oil. Season with salt and pepper.

* * *

Stuffed Crooknecks

SERVES 4

2 large yellow squash
2 tbs butter
1 3-oz cream cheese, room temperature
1 10-oz box frozen chopped spinach, thawed, drained, and squeezed dry

1 14-oz can artichoke hearts, drained and chopped
$^1/_2$ tsp lemon zest
$^1/_2$ tsp finely minced garlic
$^1/_8$ tsp cayenne pepper
salt and pepper to taste

Cut the squash lengthwise. Remove the seeds and carve out a small well. Bring a large pot of salted water to a boil and cook the squash boats for 3 minutes (tender, not mushy). Drain the boats and put them on a paper towel.

In a medium saucepan, melt the butter and the cream cheese. Use a whisk to blend. When smooth, add the remaining ingredients and stir to blend. Divide the mixture among the boats. Bake at 350°F for 25 minutes. Serve hot.

Note: You can make this into a main dish by adding 1 lb of crumbled cooked Italian sausage to the spinach mixture.

* * *

Spaghetti

SERVES 4

1 spaghetti squash
salt and pepper

butter

Cut the squash in half lengthwise. Remove the seeds and pierce the skin with a knife in several places. Spray a baking sheet with olive oil spray and lay the cut side of the squash on the sheet. Cover the squash with tinfoil. Bake for 45 minutes in a 350°F oven.

When you remove the squash from the oven, turn the flesh toward you and run a fork through it. The squash will separate into strands like spaghetti. Toss with the butter, and add salt and pepper to taste.

* * *

Tasty Cauliflower

SERVES 4 TO 6

1 head cauliflower	1/4 tsp cayenne pepper
2 tsp olive oil	1/4 cup vegetable or chicken broth
1 red pepper	1 tsp olive oil
3 cloves garlic, minced	1/4 tsp Italian seasoning

Remove the core from the cauliflower and discard. Separate the heads into flowerets. Slice the red pepper into slender strips.

Heat the 2 tsp olive oil in a skillet over medium-high heat. Sauté the flowerets, the red pepper, and the garlic for 2 minutes. Add the broth and cayenne pepper, cover the skillet, and simmer for an additional 4 minutes until the cauliflower is cooked (al dente). Remove from the heat to a serving dish, drizzle with the remaining olive oil and Italian seasoning, and add salt and pepper to taste.

* * *

Sweet Potato Cakes

SERVES 6 TO 8

3 cups mashed sweet potato	salt and pepper to taste
2 well-beaten eggs	2 tbs butter
3 tbs minced parsley	

Mix all ingredients well. Form into small cakes. Heat a medium nonstick skillet and add the butter. When it is foaming, add the potato pancakes. Let them fry until the bottoms are a golden brown (check by lifting up the cake with a spatula, but do not turn it until the bottom has browned). Repeat on the other side and serve.

* * *

The next sets of recipes are soups and appetizers that can turn any meal into a true feast. These also can make for a fun dinner party. It will be possible to entertain and to go out and enjoy yourself while following this program. These few recipes will most certainly illustrate that for you.

SOUPS AND APPETIZERS

Cucumber Soup
SERVES 4 TO 6

4 large cucumbers, seeded and
   chopped
$1/_3$ cup mint, torn
1 pinch fresh dill

1 cube chicken bouillon, dissolved
   in $1/_4$ cup of hot water
$1/_2$ cup cream
$1/_2$ cup water

Put all ingredients into a blender and whirl. The soup should be quite smooth. Refrigerate until cold. Serve garnished with a sprig of fresh mint or fresh dill.

＊ ＊ ＊

Wrapped in Red
SERVES 8

2 large sweet potatoes
12 jumbo shrimp, shelled and
   deveined

$1/_2$ tsp Creole seasoning
olive oil

Peel the sweet potatoes. Using a mandolin, slice the potato lengthwise. Bring a pot of salted water to a boil. Blanch the slices of potato until they are bendable but not too soft, about 1 minute.

Lay the potato slices on a work surface. Sprinkle with the Creole seasoning and salt and lay one raw shrimp on each slice. Roll up the shrimp and secure it with a toothpick. Leave the tail of the shrimp exposed and trim any excess potato. Pour enough oil into a hot skillet to coat it. Over high heat, sauté the shrimp until the potato wrap is golden brown. Serve immediately.

＊ ＊ ＊

Bacon-Wrapped Scallops
SERVES 10 TO 12

20 jumbo scallops
20 slices of bacon (not smoked)
20 wooden skewers

salt and pepper
drizzle of olive oil

Soak the wooden skewers in water for $1/_2$ hour.

Preheat the charcoal or gas grill.

Roll each scallop in a slice of bacon and secure the roll with a skewer. Season with salt and pepper and drizzle with olive oil. Cook over medium-high heat until almost opaque, about 4 minutes per side.

❀ ❀ ❀

Babe's Artichokes

SERVES 4

4 large artichokes	2 bunches parsley
4 cloves garlic, cut in slices	olive oil

Prepare the artichokes by slicing off each top. Slice off the stems so you have a flat bottom. With kitchen shears, trim each exposed leaf so the tip is flat. Rap the artichoke on a counter surface to loosen the globe.

Separate the leaves at the core and stuff some parsley and garlic down toward the heart. Randomly stuff parsley and garlic between the layers of the artichoke. Place the artichokes in a large pot. Drizzle the artichokes with olive oil, and season with salt and pepper. Pour water over the artichokes until water reaches about $1/_3$ up the side of the artichoke. Cover and bring the water to a gentle boil. Cook for about 40 minutes or until you can pluck a leaf easily from the artichoke. Serve warm.

❀ ❀ ❀

Onion and Sage Custards

SERVES 6

2 pounds yellow onions, sliced very thinly	2 tbs fresh sage, finely chopped
3 slices thick bacon, diced finely	1 cup heavy cream
2 tbs butter	3 large eggs
$1/_2$ tsp salt	1 tbs brown rice flour

In a large heavy saucepan, cook the bacon until crisp. With a slotted spoon, remove the bacon to some paper towels. Add the onion rings to the bacon fat and cook, stirring often until the onions are a rich brown. This will take up to 40 minutes. If the onions are too dry, add up to 2 tbs butter. When the onions are golden, sprinkle the flour over the onions and stir until the flour dissolves. Add the chopped sage and the reserved bacon and stir.

In a separate bowl, whisk the eggs until they are well mixed, and then whisk the cream into the eggs. Season with salt and pepper. Add the onions to the egg mixture and stir to combine.

Spray 6 custard cups with olive oil. Divide the onion mixture among the 6 cups and put them in a roasting pan. Fill the roasting pan with water to reach $1/2$ up the sides of the cups. Bake the custards at 350°F for 40 minutes or until the custard is well set. Serve hot.

❅ ❅ ❅

Autumn Medley Soup
SERVES 8 TO 12

2 lb red-fleshed sweet potatoes (yams)	$1/8$ tsp white pepper
1 lb butternut squash	pinch nutmeg
1 onion	1 3-oz package cream cheese, room temperature
1 tbs fresh thyme, minced	3 tbs heavy cream
1 tbs fresh sage, minced	1 tsp fresh thyme
2 tbs olive oil	1 tbs fresh sage
5 cups chicken broth	

Peel the sweet potatoes and cut them into 1-inch cubes. Cut the butternut in half and scoop out the seeds and strings. Peel the squash and cut it into 1-inch cubes. Peel the onion and quarter it. Assemble these vegetables and the herbs in a roasting pan. Add the olive oil and toss the vegetables until they are evenly coated. Roast in a 400°F oven for 45 minutes. Stir the mixture every 15 minutes to prevent sticking and to encourage even browning.

Purée the vegetables in a blender, adding the chicken stock as needed. Transfer to a soup pot and heat thoroughly. Ladle into soup bowls and garnish with a dollop of herb cream.

Herb cream: In the bowl of a food processor fitted with a steel blade, mince the herbs. Add the cream cheese and cream, and process until smooth. It should be thick but pourable. Add additional cream if needed.

❅ ❅ ❅

Black Bean Soup with Avocado Salsa
SERVES 8 TO 12

1 lb black beans	2 cloves garlic, minced
2 tbs macadamia nut oil	$1/4$ tsp cayenne pepper
2 large onions, diced	1 bay leaf (not Californian)
2 ribs celery, diced	8 cups ham or chicken stock

Pick over the beans and remove any that have gone bad. Cover the good beans with cold water and allow them to soak overnight.

In a soup pot, heat the macadamia nut oil. Add the onions, celery, and garlic, and sauté until soft. Add the beans, bay leaf, cayenne, and stock. Simmer until the beans are soft and breaking up. Transfer in batches to a blender. Process the soup to your liking, either with chunks of beans or totally puréed. Return to the pot to reheat. Check seasonings, and add salt and pepper as need. Serve with a dollop of avocado salsa in the center.

* * *

Avocado Salsa for Black Bean Soup

2 avocados, ripe, peeled, and cut into $1/_2$-inch dice
$1/_4$ cup cilantro, minced

5 radishes, sliced as thinly as possible
2 tbs fresh lime juice

Combine all ingredients; add salt and pepper as needed. Serve immediately with black bean soup.

* * *

15

A Resource Guide

There are many organizations that can give you a wealth of information about your disease. I am going to list these in no particular order. I am also going to include places where you can find out more information about the food sensitivity testing and some of the other testing that your doctor may not be so familiar with. I will list them under the heading "Complementary Medical Information."

General Medical Information

Asthma and Allergy Foundation of America
    1233 20th Street NW, Suite 402
    Washington, DC 20036
    800-727-8462
    info@aafa.org
    www.aafa.org

This organization is dedicated to improving the quality of life for people with asthma and allergies. They publish *Advance*, a bimonthly consumer newsletter; they also have a special Web page for kids and teens.

American Lung Association
  1740 Broadway
  New York, NY 10019
  800-586-4872
  www.lungusa.org
  info@lungusa.org

Detailed information is provided about asthma, events, publications, and links on their Web site. This is the official party line site.

National Institute of Allergy and Infectious Disease
  NIAID Office of Communication and Public Liaison
  31 Center Drive MSC 2520
  Building 31, Room 7A-50
  Bethesda, MD 20892-2520
  www.niaid.nih.org

Food and Drug Administration
  Office of Consumer Affairs/HFE-88
  5600 Fishers Lane
  Rockville, MD 20857
  888-463-6332
  www.fda.gov

This site provides information about allergies that you may find helpful.

American College of Allergy, Asthma, and Immunology
  85 West Algonquin Road, Suite 550
  Arlington Heights, IL 60005
  800-842-7777
  www.allergy.mcg.edu

American Academy of Allergy, Asthma, and Immunology
  611 East Wells Street
  Milwaukee, WI 53202
  414-272-6071
  www.aaaai.org

National Institute of Environmental Health Sciences
  Office of Communications
  P.O. Box 12233
  Research Triangle Park, NC 27709
  919-541-3345
  www.niehs.nih.gov/airborne/prevent/intro.html

This site gives good information about local allergens and offers prevention strategies for seasonal afflictions.

Allergy and Asthma Network
   Mothers of Asthmatics, Inc.
   2751 Prosperity Avenue, Suite 150
   Fairfax, VA 22031
   703-641-9595
   www.aanma.org

The Food Allergy and Anaphylaxis Network
   10400 Eaton Place, Suite 107
   Fairfax, VA 22030
   800-929-4040
   www.foodallergy.org

This site will give you information on true food allergies.

The following URL is for children and provides diagrams of the respiratory system and easy-to-understand information and illustrations of causes and symptoms of asthma:

www.people.virginia.edu/~smb4v/tutorials/asthma/asthma1.html

The addresses and sites listed above are all highly conventional in their thinking. Some of these sites may even tell you that most of what I have just told you is all wrong. As I said, they can have their opinion and I can have mine. I think that some of these sites do contain valuable information if you just learn to take the information you need and ignore the rhetoric.

Complementary Medical Information

American College of Advancement in Medicine (ACAM)
   P.O. Box 3427
   Laguna Hills, CA 92654
   800-532-3688
   www.acam.org

This is an organization that can refer you to a doctor in your area who practices the same type of medicine I do.

International and American Associations of Clinical Nutritionists
   16775 Addison Road, Suite 100
   Addison, TX 75001
   972-407-9089
   www.iaacn.org

This is an organization that holds the same food beliefs I do—that the right foods can help heal you. They can help you find a nutritionist in your area if you can't find or don't want another doctor.

Doctor's Data, Inc., and Reference Laboratory
    3755 Illinois Ave.
    St. Charles, IL 60174-2420
    708-231-3649
    www.doctorsdata.com

They provide many of the laboratory tests I discuss in this book.

Great Smokies Diagnostic Laboratory
    63 Zillicoa Street
    Asheville, NC 28806
    828-253-0621
    www.greatsmokies.lab.com

They also provide the testing.

Meta Metrix Medical Laboratory
    5000 Peachtree Industrial Boulevard, Suite 110
    Norcross, GA 30071
    800-221-4640
    www.metametrix.com

They also provide the testing.

AMTL Corporation
    One Oakwood Boulevard, Suite 130
    Hollywood, FL 33020
    954-923-2990

They do the food sensitivity test I perform most often on my patients.

Each of the above laboratories would be happy to help you locate a practitioner in your area who can do the testing.

To get in contact with me, please write or call:

Fred Pescatore, M.D., M.P.H.
    Dana Cohen, M.D.
    274 Madison Avenue, Suite 402
    New York, NY 10016
    212-779-2944

To find out more information about weight-loss programs or Dr. Pescatore's complete line of Healthy for Good Food Products, please contact:

Thin For Good Weight Loss Centers
274 Madison Avenue, Suite 402
New York, NY 10016
888-350-8446 (THIN)
www.thinforgood.com
www.macnutoil.com

Index

Printed in the USA
CPSIA information can be obtained
at www.ICGtesting.com
LVHW091512080824
787695LV00001B/68

9 780470 275412